Resynchronization and Defibrillation for Heart Failure

A Practical Approach

Resynchronization and Defibrillation for Heart Failure

A Practical Approach

Editors

David L. Hayes, MD
Paul J. Wang, MD
Jonathan Sackner-Bernstein, MD
Samuel J. Asirvatham, MD

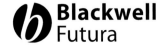

Published by Blackwell Publishing, 9600 Garsington Road, Oxford OX4 2DQ, UK

Printed and bound by Narayana Press, in Denmark.

Care has been taken to confirm the accuracy of the information presented and to describe generally accepted practices. However, the authors, editors, and publisher are not responsible for errors or omissions or for any consequences from application of the information in this book and make no warranty, express or implied, with respect to the contents of the publication. This book should not be relied on apart from the advice of a qualified health care provider.

The authors, editors, and publisher have exerted efforts to ensure that drug selection and dosage set forth in this text are in accordance with current recommendations and practice at the time of publication. However, in view of ongoing research, changes in government regulations, and the constant flow of information relating to drug therapy and drug reactions, the reader is urged to check the package insert for each drug for any change in indications and dosage and for added warnings and precautions. This is particularly important when the recommended agent is a new or infrequently employed drug.

Some drugs and medical devices presented in this publication have U.S. Food and Drug Administration (FDA) clearance for limited use in restricted research settings. It is the responsibility of health care providers to ascertain the FDA status of each drug or device planned for use in their clinical practice.

ISBN: 1-4051-2199-8

Library of Congress Cataloging-in-Publication Data

Resynchronization and defibrillation for heart failure : a practical approach / editors, David L. Hayes ... [et al.].-- 1st ed.
   p. ; cm.
 Includes bibliographical references and index.
 ISBN 1-4051-2199-8 (hard cover : alk. paper)
 1. Heart failure--Treatment. 2. Cardiac pacing. 3. Electric countershock. 4. Arrhythmia--Treatment.
 [DNLM: 1. Heart Failure, Congestive--therapy. 2. Arrhythmia--therapy. 3. Cardiac Pacing, Artificial. 4. Defibrillators, Implantable. 5. Pacemaker, Artificial. 6. Ventricular Dysfunction--therapy. WG 370 R436 2004] I. Hayes, David L. II. Title.

 RC685.C53R47 2004
 616.1'2906--dc22

                                2004000363

Catalogue records are also available from The British Library.

DEDICATION

To our wives and families

ACKNOWLEDGMENTS

The authors would like to acknowledge the staff of the Mayo Clinic Section of Scientific Publications, without which this book would not be possible. Although many in the section contributed to this work, several should be individually acknowledged for having invested many hours of their time: Sharon Wadleigh, for layout, typing, and attention to many details; O. Eugene Millhouse, Ph.D., for editing; Kenna Atherton, for proofreading; and Roberta Schwartz, for her general publishing expertise and not allowing any obstacles to get in the way of seeing the book to fruition. The authors also want to acknowledge the staff in Media Support Services, particularly Jeff Satre, for art direction and book design; John Hagen, for the cover illustration; and their colleagues Alice McKinney, medical illustrator; Jim Tidwell and Bryce Bergene, scientific illustrators; and Peggy Chehak, digital artist. This is truly a phenomenal group of individuals, and we have been very fortunate to have this "team."

We would also like to acknowledge the many individuals who have contributed to the body of literature that has become "cardiac resynchronization therapy." Many of these pioneers are referenced in the text and are to be congratulated for helping to advance this rapidly evolving discipline.

AUTHOR AFFILIATIONS

David L. Hayes, M.D.
>   Chair, Division of Cardiovascular Diseases and Internal
>   Medicine, Mayo Clinic; Professor of Medicine, Mayo Clinic
>   College of Medicine; Rochester, Minnesota

Paul J. Wang, M.D.
>   Director, Stanford Cardiac Arrhythmia Services & Cardiac
>   Electrophysiology Laboratories, Stanford University Medical
>   Center; Professor of Medicine, Stanford University School of
>   Medicine; Stanford, California

Jonathan Sackner-Bernstein, M.D.
>   Director, Heart Failure Prevention and Treatment Clinic;
>   Director, Clinical Research, Clinical Scholars Program, Heart
>   Failure and Cardiomyopathy Center, North Shore University
>   Hospital; Manhasset, New York

Samuel J. Asirvatham, M.D.
>   Senior Associate Consultant, Division of Cardiovascular
>   Diseases and Internal Medicine, Mayo Clinic; Assistant
>   Professor of Medicine, Mayo Clinic College of Medicine;
>   Rochester, Minnesota

CONTRIBUTING AUTHOR

Theodore P. Abraham, M.D.
>   Senior Associate Consultant, Division of Cardiovascular
>   Diseases and Internal Medicine, Mayo Clinic; Assistant
>   Professor of Medicine, Mayo Clinic College of Medicine;
>   Rochester, Minnesota

TABLE OF CONTENTS

Introduction

The motivation for this text was the clinical challenge of understanding and applying the rapidly evolving new discipline of device therapy for heart failure. In some ways, it is unprecedented that two sub-subspecialty areas should become so "co-dependent." All five of us who wrote this book practice in academic centers, where we operate within fairly strict sub-subspecialties of cardiology. We come from the disciplines of implantable device therapy (D.L.H., P.J.W., S.J.A.), electrophysiology (P.J.W., S.J.A.), echocardiography (T.P.A.), and heart failure management (J.S.-B.). Before beginning to write this book, we understood that we had much to learn from one another, as we since have, and thought that our individual skills would be complementary in preparing a "blended" approach to device therapy for heart failure management. We realize that many cardiologists actively practice—and are expert in—both implantable device therapy and heart failure management. We also are aware that many internists and generalists are expert in heart failure management.

Our hope is that this text will provide a foundation for increased understanding of device therapy for patients suffering from ventricular dysfunction and heart failure. The text is intended to provide insight into the basic areas of device therapy, heart failure management, and sudden cardiac death. Readers who are expert in one or two of these areas will be able to acquire basic information about the other area or areas. We hope that readers whose scope of practice already envelopes all three areas will benefit from the new clinical arena that arises from combining these disciplines. It is too early in the experience to know who will eventually assume the responsibility of managing patients after cardiac resynchronization therapy. If this area of cardiology evolves like any other, it will probably be dependent on many factors, including the type of practice, the location of the practice, the desires of the patient, referral patterns, and reimbursement issues. In contrast, the management of patients with implanted defibrillators is well defined, although variability remains because of the factors cited above. Interrogation of the defibrillator requires specific tools and training, and similar skill levels most likely will be needed to interrogate and program biventricular pacemakers.

With the rapid evolution of device therapy for heart failure and constant redefinition of what is "state of the art," we are bound by some limitations. Several clinical trials are still under way, and data are not available or are very preliminary. Other clinical trials have been completed, but the results have not been published in articles. Information from these trials may be available as abstracted data, but other information has been presented only in "late-breaking" trial sessions at national meetings and is not even available in abstract form. Also, data from the prospective trials are protected until they are published in a peer-reviewed journal.

There are also limitations of knowledge in the area. As in any newer discipline, understanding one facet of the application leads to many more questions. Because of this evolutionary process, which is rapid in comparison with progress in many areas, we see this text as only a beginning. We look forward to providing updates to this text in our effort to share both the results of further investigations and the practical aspects of the application to clinical practice. In the final chapter of the book, we also look to the future and discuss the questions that are currently being asked, the investigations under way to answer them, and the technologies and therapies that may eventually eclipse device therapy for heart failure as we now know it.

CHAPTER 1

What Is Heart Failure and What Are The Treatment Options? Complex Questions

Jonathan Sackner-Bernstein, MD

A patient was presented on morning rounds. The resident said the patient was admitted *for* heart failure, responded to therapy, and now was no longer *in* heart failure. What is meant by "admitted *for* heart failure" and "no longer *in* heart failure?" Did the patient necessarily have impaired ventricular function? Now that the patient no longer had failure, how aggressive should treatment be? Although these questions may seem mundane, the answers frame the approach to the patient and determine the clinical course.

Traditionally, heart failure was considered a state of fluid overload that was treated by management of the congestion. The terms "*in* heart failure" and "*out* of heart failure" came to reflect volume status and were commonly applied to any patient who had volume overload, including those with congestion caused by renal failure, liver failure, or pure right-heart failure due to pulmonary vascular disease. Because the management for each of these conditions is quite different, diagnostic testing is required whenever heart disease is suspected as a cause of fluid retention.[1-4] In each of these conditions, the underlying pathophysiologic mechanism leading to clinical progression needs to be treated, not merely the state of congestion. For this reason, thinking of a patient as being "in" or "out of" heart failure provides a false sense of security. Even when volume status is optimal, the risk of disease progression is high, and the first manifestation of progression can be sudden cardiac death.[1] Therefore, physicians must choose medications and devices that reduce this risk of death as well as improve the quality of life.

Why do physicians focus on congestion? The traditional view of heart failure as a state of congestion is reinforced by the episodes of fluid retention that prompt many office visits and hospitalizations. However, fluid retention is a relatively late manifestation of the disease, appearing after ventricular function has deteriorated markedly and perhaps irreversibly. At this stage, the disease has already become a systemic illness, and various neurohormonal systems that accelerate the disease process have been activated. Waiting for the manifestation of fluid retention instead of providing treatment in the early stages of ventricular dysfunction can be compared to waiting for a patient to present with metastatic cancer instead of screening for a primary tumor. The primary focus of this book is the treatment of heart failure utilizing device therapy. Also, in following the new staging system for heart failure developed by the American Heart Association (AHA) and the American College of Cardiology (ACC),[3] the clinical focus must include all patients who are at risk for developing heart failure and those with impaired ventricular function, whether symptomatic or not (Table 1).

Reviews of the pathophysiology and treatment of heart failure have described the factors that lead to disease progression and the importance of proven therapies.[1-5] This chapter considers perspectives that are complementary to these reviews and, in many ways, are more crucial for achieving optimal management of patients with heart failure (Table 2). First, overt heart failure is the end result of progressive ventricular dysfunction, and data support the use of medications very early in the process, including the treatment of patients with asymptomatic left ventricular dysfunction.[5] Second, heart failure should be suspected and screened for,[1-4] similar to the approach used for colorectal and other cancers. Third, heart failure is a disease that affects people even when their volume status is optimal. Fourth, despite a desire to learn of a new breakthrough in the management of heart failure, one that will cure the disease, the breakthrough is already at our fingertips, with therapies proven to prevent and reverse the severity of heart failure, primarily angiotensin-converting enzyme (ACE) inhibitors[6-13] and β-blockers,[14-19] with an emerging role for aldosterone antagonism.[20,21] Fifth, device therapy of heart failure can improve the quality of life and decrease the risk of death when used in conjunction with medical therapy.[22-26]

Table 1. Stages of Heart Failure According to AHA/ACC Guidelines

Stage	Description
A	Patients at high risk (hypertension, coronary artery disease, diabetes mellitus, positive family history)
B	Patients with structural heart disease but without signs or symptoms of heart failure
C	Patients who have current or previous symptoms of heart failure associated with underlying structural heart disease
D	Patients with structural heart disease and marked symptoms of heart failure at rest despite maximal therapy

ACC, American College of Cardiology; AHA, American Heart Association.
Modified from Hunt et al.[3] By permission of the American Heart Association.

Table 2. List of the Key Perspectives

Heart failure is a predictable process, start medical therapy early
Heart failure is detectable early, providing opportunity to reduce morbidity and
  mortality
Patients still have heart failure after congestion has resolved
ACE inhibitors and β-blockers, used more widely, are powerful tools against the
  disease (as are aldosterone antagonists and, in selected cases, ARBs)
Device therapy provides additional benefit, with little morbidity to patients

ACE, angiotensin-converting enzyme; ARB, angiotensin receptor blocker.

Standard treatment of heart failure and ventricular dysfunction includes ACE inhibitors,[6-13] β-blockers,[14-17,19] and aldosterone antagonists,[20,21] with additional benefit from digoxin[27] and diuretics.[28] Statins and antithrombotic therapy can prevent infarcts[29-31] and the development of heart failure[32] in those at risk. The use of defibrillators[22,25] and biventricular pacemakers,[24] potentially simultaneously,[26,33] improves the quality of life and reduces the risk of death.

Epidemiology of Heart Failure:
Classic Description Does Not Tell the Whole Story

When epidemiologists report that 5 million Americans are affected by heart failure,[1-4] they refer to patients with symptomatic disease. Random screening in the United Kingdom showed a striking incidence of asymptomatic left ventricular dysfunction, especially in persons between the ages of 45 and 65 years.[34] This suggests that asymptomatic left ventricular dysfunction likely affects several million people more than the 5 million with heart failure reported by epidemiologists.

With such a large number of patients having asymptomatic left ventricular dysfunction and thus being at risk for death, including an increased risk of sudden death,[35] the approach to the detection of disease must change. The incidence of symptomatic heart failure in the Framingham cohort is markedly higher than that of colon cancer for persons older than 50 years (Fig. 1). This disparity would be even greater if the incidence of asymptomatic left ventricular dysfunction were included. With therapies able to slow the progression of disease from hypertension and coronary artery disease to left ventricular dysfunction and, ultimately, symptomatic heart failure, screening for and treating these early stages should be part of standard care. Despite the economic cost, the obligation to patients is to ensure that they are evaluated for diseases that pose significant risk and they receive treatment that can safely and effectively reduce that risk.

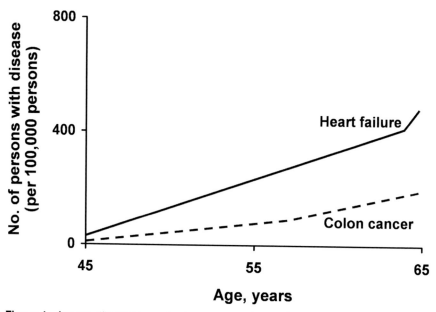

Figure 1. Age-specific incidence of colon cancer and stage C or D heart failure. (Data from Kannel WB, Belanter AJ. Epidemiology of heart failure. Am Heart J 1991;121:951-7 and the National Cancer Institute. SEER Incidence & US Mortality Statistics. Available at http://seer.cancer.gov/canques/. Accessed October 23, 2003.)

In the 1970s, the American Cancer Society realized that the likelihood of colorectal cancer increased markedly in persons older than 50 years. This observation led to the conclusion that persons older than 50 were at average risk and required flexible sigmoidoscopy every 5 years or colonoscopy every 10 years in addition to fecal occult blood testing.[36,37] If a patient has additional risk factors, including a positive family history, the screening strategy intensifies.

Data from the Framingham Heart Study show a similar increase in risk of heart failure for persons older than 50 years. However, the magnitude of this risk is much higher than that for colorectal cancer (Fig. 1).[38] The Framingham data also point to several factors that increase the risk of structural changes to the left ventricle: the presence of coronary artery disease, hypertension, diabetes mellitus, and valvular lesions.[39,40] Individually, these factors markedly increase the risk of heart failure for both men and women. The most important fact is that if heart failure is not suspected clinically, the diagnosis will not be made until late in the clinical course, by which time the patients who are fortunate will be suffering and others will have had sudden cardiac death. For these reasons, patients in this high-risk group who have abnormal ventricular geometry or function need to be identified and therapy initiated immediately.

Although this recommendation may be unexpected, consider the basis for screening for colorectal cancer with flexible sigmoidoscopy or colonoscopy in patients beginning at age 50. In 2001, the American Cancer Society estimated that fewer than 150,000 cases of colorectal cancer would be diagnosed.[38] Considering that the risk of heart failure is at least comparable to that of colorectal cancer, that available therapies can reduce disease progression and the risk of sudden death, and that the number of patients affected is large, heart failure warrants similar aggressiveness in diagnostic strategies. The population at risk for heart failure can be drawn from a well-recognized group of patients, namely, those with coronary artery disease, hypertension, or diabetes mellitus, especially those older than 50 years. The diagnosis of ventricular dysfunction mandates treatment with ACE inhibitors, β-blockers, and, potentially, defibrillators for patients with coronary artery disease and a low ejection fraction who have nonsustained ventricular tachycardia. The use of these treatments could decrease the risk of death by more than 50%.[41]

A proactive detection strategy for patients who have identifiable risk factors would seem prudent, but it appears to be contrary to published guidelines. However, published guidelines state that patients in whom heart failure is suspected should undergo testing to determine whether cardiac function is abnormal. Suspicion should be raised when a patient presents with dyspnea, fatigue, or signs of congestion, including rales, hepatic congestion, ascites, or dependent edema. However, a large body of literature indicates that several other factors can identify patients earlier in the disease process and lead to evaluation. These factors include the presence of coronary artery disease, diabetes, hypertension or valvular disease,[1] and age older than 50 years (Fig. 1). Published guidelines describe the diagnostic pursuit for reversible causes of heart failure[1-3]; a review of these issues is beyond the scope of this monograph.

Investigating for evidence of exercise intolerance, whether by formal testing or detailed history taking, is the best way to diagnose symptomatic heart failure, even when volume status is optimal. Patients generally consider a reduction in exercise capacity as a sign of aging, and specific and aggressive inquiry is required to detect a clinically meaningful change. Waiting for the disease to become symptomatic before starting aggressive medical therapy may expose patients to greater risk than necessary.

Another technique that has been advocated for detecting ventricular dysfunction is measurement of natriuretic peptides; however, the utility of the assay for brain natriuretic peptide has been assessed primarily in patients who present with dyspnea or other signs or symptoms that suggest decompensated heart failure.[42,43] For these patients, echocardiography is recommended by the current treatment guidelines.[1-4] The brain natriuretic peptide assay appears useful in titrating the intensity of treatment in patients with established heart failure.[44]

The strategy for proactively identifying patients with stage A or B heart failure closely parallels those published by several organizations for the detection and management of various cancers. Once caregivers become sensitive to suspecting a structural abnormality, in this case ventricular dysfunction, we must screen for the lesion and treat it aggressively with ACE inhibitors and β-blockers. Hyperlipidemia, hypertension, and diabetes should be treated to meet the strictest goals. Patients should be considered candidates for defibrillators[22,25] and resynchronization therapy[24,26,33] after medical therapy has been optimized, in accordance with the practices in clinical trials.

Prognosis of Heart Failure

Prevention becomes more important when the prognosis of the disease is considered. Epidemiologic databases indicate that the prognosis for patients who present with heart failure is dismal: one-half die within 2 to 3 years after the diagnosis is made (Fig. 2). This may have improved statistically but not in a clinically impressive fashion (Fig. 3).[45]

These data are in marked contrast to the risk reported by randomized controlled trials. For example, patients rendered asymptomatic with ACE inhibitor and

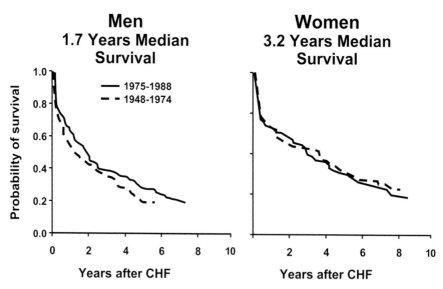

Figure 2. Newly diagnosed congestive heart failure (CHF) requiring hospitalization is high risk for men and women (the Framingham experience). (From Ho KK, Anderson KM, Kannel WB, Grossman W, Levy D. Survival after the onset of congestive heart failure in Framingham Heart Study subjects. Circulation 1993;88:107-15. By permission of the American Heart Association.)

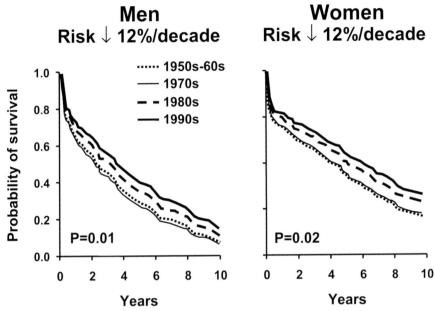

Figure 3. Clinical outcomes with heart failure in the Framingham study improved statistically, but without marked clinical impact. (Modified from Levy et al.[45] By permission of the Massachusetts Medical Society.)

β-blocker therapy despite left ventricular dysfunction after a myocardial infarction have less than a 5% risk of death within 1 year,[46] compared with the 25% risk reported elsewhere.[35] In the Carvedilol or Metoprolol European Trial (COMET), a trial of patients in New York Heart Association (NYHA) functional class II or III, the annual mortality rate of those receiving ACE inhibitor and β-blocker therapy was 8%,[17] compared with the median survival of less than 3 years for the Framingham cohort.[45] These differences are ascribed largely to patient selection and close follow-up in the clinical trials. Clinical trials attempt to study a population affected only by the disease of interest, in this case, heart failure. Therefore, patients who have heart failure but severe renal insufficiency may be excluded. For example, a typical limit for serum creatinine may be 2.5 to 3.0 mg/dL. As for follow-up, most clinical trials include centers with research nurses involved in ongoing case management, a technique that is not available in most clinical practices. Case management of patients with heart failure markedly reduces hospitalizations and is associated with improved quality of life.[47]

Talking to a patient about the risks becomes difficult when faced with uncertainty about quantifying prognosis. Generally, discussing the traditional view and comparing it with the recent clinical trial data can serve to indicate the severity of the condition while providing hope. Patients usually ask questions in a way that reveals how much information they want to hear; listening for these cues can make the educational process more useful. Because of the nature of the disease, it is important to address end-of-life wishes without forcing the issue.[48] It can be revisited later. Because the course of the disease depends on patient compliance and cooperation, providing patients with a reason for a positive outlook is important.

Ventricular Remodeling

Ventricular dysfunction occurs as part of the process of ventricular remodeling, which refers to the change in the shape, structure, and function of the ventricle that is the hallmark of disease progression. The process starts when the myocardium is affected by an injury, which can be abrupt in onset or chronic (Fig. 4).[49]

Clinically, the progressive course of ventricular remodeling varies somewhat with the cause. Although a review of the molecular and cellular aspects of remodeling[50] is beyond the intended scope of this book, the process can be summarized for the two most common causes of heart failure, namely, ischemic and hypertensive heart disease. After myocardial infarction, the noninfarcted myocardium

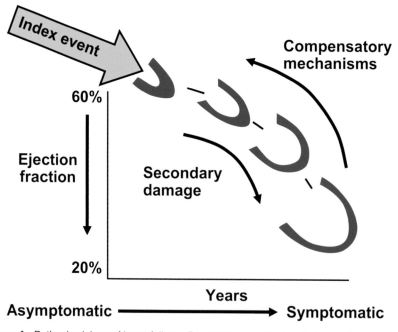

Figure 4. Pathophysiology of heart failure. Progressive ventricular dilation and dysfunction lead to progressive symptoms. (From Mann.[49] By permission of the American Heart Association.)

compensates to maintain chamber performance. These segments immediately become hypercontractile and begin to hypertrophy. Subsequently, they are exposed to greater workloads and greater wall stress, which trigger the release of neurohormones and cytokines that lead to cellular dysfunction and death through apoptosis.[51] The viable myocytes elongate (cellular remodeling), physiologically driven by an effort to reduce the hemodynamic stress on the individual cells. However, the net effect is a globular, dilated, hypocontractile ventricle.

In contrast, patients with hypertension develop concentric left ventricular hypertrophy, thus reducing the stress on each myocyte. In this case, the compensatory mechanism reduces the workload on individual cells but leads to myocardial fibrosis and diastolic stiffening of the ventricle, exacerbating the increased filling pressures. Eventually, these hemodynamic forces cause increased wall stress and the release of neurohormones and cytokines that lead to the development of a globular and dilated hypocontractile left ventricle indistinguishable from that of end-stage heart failure due to ischemic heart disease.

Once the process of remodeling starts, the natural history leads inevitably to heart failure, unless sudden death occurs. Also, the extent of remodeling,[52,53] and the extent to which it can be reversed by therapy, correlates with outcome.[52,54] The consistency of this relationship allows the identification of patients at risk and the introduction of antiremodeling therapies (ACE inhibitors, β-blockers, and aldosterone antagonists).[20,21] The opportunity for impact is substantial, with only 65% to 70% of patients receiving treatment with ACE inhibitors or β-blockers.[25] If 90% of patients were treated, thousands of lives would be saved.

Lifestyle

Success with any therapeutic strategy is enhanced markedly with patient education. Patients who have heart failure must understand salt restriction, avoidance of toxins (tobacco, drugs, and excess alcohol), and the value of routine exercise. By making patients partners, their role in watching for signs and symptoms of worsening heart failure enables physicians to be more effective with treatment because physicians know about problems early in the presentation. For example, a female patient weighs herself daily and notices a 2- to 3-lb weight gain over 2 or 3 days. She may or may not recall dietary sodium indiscretion but likely does not feel any worsening of her symptoms. If nothing is done, she probably will feel worse in a few days and end up in the emergency department within a week. Instead, the physician can instruct her to double her diuretic dose for a day. In most cases, she will call the next day to report that she feels fine and her weight is back to its previous level. This is not possible unless the patient understands surveillance strategies and knows how to contact the physician. The two keys for making a patient a partner in care are an open channel for communication and insight into the management plan.

As an extension of this approach, suggesting specific resources to patients can markedly enhance their understanding and participation in the care plan.[55]

Medical Therapy

Neurohormonal antagonists reverse ventricular remodeling, slow the progression of heart failure, improve symptoms, and reduce the risk of death.[6-8,10,14-16,18,19,28,46,56] All patients with heart failure should receive at least two neurohormonal antagonists: ACE inhibitors and β-blockers. Clinical trial data interpreted within the pathophysiologic mechanisms of the disease support the use of ACE inhibitors and β-blockers for patients with stage A disease to prevent disease progression and reduce the risk of death.[12,57]

For patients with stage C or D disease, device-based therapy should be considered after the medical regimen has been optimized. Although many advocate the use of vasodilators, for example, hydralazine and isosorbide,[58] they are unproven therapies. The data regarding angiotensin receptor blockers are not completely concordant. Valsartan appears to increase risk when added to β-blockers and ACE inhibitors. However, this may be only a statistical anomaly.[59] In contrast, the Candesartan Heart Failure Assessment of Reduction in Mortality and Morbidity (CHARM) study demonstrated consistent benefit of candesartan in patients with heart failure independent of background therapy or ejection fraction.[60]

Treating Heart Failure as More Than a State of Congestion

Heart failure cannot be viewed merely as a state of intermittent congestion surrounding periods of clinical stability. The notion that treatment that produces a compensated state is sufficient is incorrect. This does not mean that all patients can achieve a truly asymptomatic state, NYHA class I, with treatment but rather that mere improvement in fluid status and symptoms is not satisfactory. Patients whose condition appears "stable" remain at high risk for disease progression, including the possibility that the first manifestation of disease progression may be sudden death. For this reason, treatment with ACE inhibitors, β-blockers, and, when appropriate, aldosterone antagonists and angiotensin receptor blockers in addition to the use of devices (discussed in subsequent chapters) need to be part of the clinical strategy for all patients with ventricular dysfunction and heart failure.

Adrenergic Antagonists

Clinical Trials

Adrenergic antagonism is standard care for patients with heart failure (Fig. 5). β-Blockers reduce symptoms, slow disease progression, and decrease the risk of

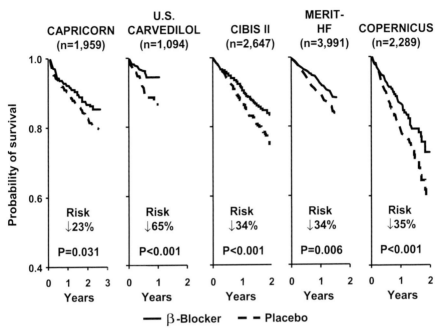

Figure 5. β-Blockers reduce the risk of death for patients with left ventricular dysfunction after myocardial infarction and those with symptomatic heart failure (Stages B through D).[14-16,19,46] (From Sackner-Bernstein J, Kelly K. Before it happens to you: a breakthrough program for reversing or preventing heart disease. Cambridge, MA, Da Capo Press, 2004. Copyrighted by and used with permission from Jonathan Sackner-Bernstein, MD.)

death.[14-16,19,61] They are effective for heart failure of ischemic or nonischemic cause[14,15,19] and improve outcome whether patients are minimally symptomatic or have advanced disease.[14-16,19,46,61] However, not all agents that antagonize the sympathetic nervous system have the same effect.[16,62,63] Therefore, it cannot be assumed that all adrenergic antagonists are interchangeable for the treatment of heart failure, and in the climate of evidence-based medicine, the agents proven to be effective in randomized controlled clinical trials should be selected. The β-blockers currently available differ in their specificity for β_1- and β_2-receptors, and some (e.g., metoprolol and bisoprolol) are considered relatively β_1-receptor selective and others (e.g., carvedilol) relatively nonselective. Recent data suggest that metoprolol may be less β_1 selective than previously considered. In a controlled trial that compared carvedilol with metoprolol succinate, patients had doses titrated toward the target and at each visit β_2 antagonism was assessed by measuring glucose and potassium during the infusion of terbutaline. This study demonstrated that 100 mg of metoprolol succinate is mildly selective and 200 mg is not selective at all relative to carvedilol 12.5 and 25 mg bid, respectively.[64] Several β-blockers also have other pharmacologic properties; for example, carvedilol has α_1-blocking (vasodilator) and antioxidant properties and bucindolol also causes vasodilation, although the mechanism is not clear. Until recently, it was not known whether these pharmacologic differences resulted in clinically meaningful differences. Although three β-blockers—carvedilol, metoprolol, and bisoprolol—improve clinical outcome in heart failure, carvedilol is superior to metoprolol, according to the results of COMET.[17]

Drug Selection

Although the initial randomized studies that compared carvedilol and metoprolol were not sufficiently powered to show a clinical difference in outcome, the surrogate end points evaluated were intriguing.[65-68] Metra et al.[68] evaluated the effects on ventricular performance and exercise hemodynamics in 150 patients randomly assigned to carvedilol or metoprolol for up to 44 months. When reassessed after 13 to 15 months of treatment, both groups showed improvement, but the carvedilol group had a significantly greater increase in left ventricular ejection fraction at rest, left ventricular stroke volume, and stroke work during exercise and a greater decrease in mean pulmonary wedge pressure both at rest and during exercise than the metoprolol group. In contrast, the metoprolol group had a greater increase in maximal exercise capacity than the carvedilol group. Di Lenarda et al.[67] evaluated the effects of carvedilol in 30 patients who were limited by symptoms of heart failure and ventricular dysfunction after at least 1 year of treatment with metoprolol. In this open-label study, the left ventricular ejection fraction improved significantly by 1 year after treatment was changed from metoprolol to carvedilol. In contrast, two studies that randomly assigned patients to carvedilol or metoprolol found no differences in hemodynamics[65,66] or measures of oxidative stress,[65] although carvedilol significantly reduced left ventricular end-diastolic dimension to a greater extent.[66] However, the surrogates used in these studies were not necessarily predictive of clinical effects. This is even more apparent when it is appreciated that the adrenergic antagonist moxonidine decreases sympathetic activation[69] yet increases the risk of death.[62]

Carvedilol, metoprolol, and bisoprolol all improve well-being and reduce the risk of death. However, the results of COMET allow a more definitive prioritizing of the usefulness of particular β-blockers in the treatment of heart failure. COMET compared carvedilol (25 mg bid) and metoprolol tartrate (50 mg bid) and demonstrated that carvedilol reduced the risk of death significantly better than metoprolol tartrate.[17] Some may find it difficult to apply these data to clinical practice because metoprolol tartrate was studied but metoprolol succinate is the formulation proven effective for heart failure.

Despite the many ways the data can be interpreted, a simple view may be the most useful for clinical practice. Because carvedilol has proven to be better than another β-blocker and the same cannot be claimed for any other β-blocker, carvedilol must be viewed as a drug superior within its class. Perhaps another drug may prove to belong to the same category, as a superior β-blocker, but until data support this designation, carvedilol is the only one. Therefore, on the basis of the available data,[17] all patients with heart failure should receive treatment with carvedilol. Alternatively, because the decrease in heart rate with carvedilol and metoprolol tartrate was similar over the course of the study, with less than a 2-beat per minute difference, and the drugs were dosed for comparable β_1-blockade, the superiority of carvedilol may reflect the importance of β_2- and α_1-blockade.

Metabolic Effects

Carvedilol produces metabolic effects different from those of metoprolol[70] and atenolol (Fig. 6),[71] and this may be clinically relevant because of the link between insulin resistance and clinical outcomes.[72-74] The mechanism of this difference appears to be related to the α_1 antagonism of carvedilol.[75] If this effect were independent of the antihypertensive effects of these agents, it could prove important because nondiabetic patients with mild-to-moderate heart failure can be insulin-resistant.[76-79] The COMET investigators reported a lower incidence of new-onset diabetes in those treated with carvedilol compared with those treated with metoprolol (Poole-Wilson P, presented at the annual meeting of the European Society of Cardiology, Vienna, Austria, August 30 to September 2, 2003), confirming that the choice of β-blocker should be individualized.

Strategies for Clinical Practice

β-Blockers should be administered to all patients with symptomatic heart failure when their condition is stabilized with oral medications[1,2,16] as well as to patients with left ventricular dysfunction after myocardial infarction.[46] Background therapy should include diuretics as required, digoxin, and ACE inhibitors. This strategy could be extended to asymptomatic patients who have only mild left ventricular dysfunction, on the basis of data from patients treated after myocardial infarction[46] (stage B heart failure), the known pathophysiologic mechanism of the disease,[80] and the risk that the first manifestation of disease progression can be sudden death.

Patients with severe heart failure who require inotropic agents intravenously or other assist devices should start receiving β-blocker therapy when weaned from intravenous medications and stabilized on oral agents.[16] The starting doses of β-blockers should be as low as possible, with a gradual increase over several weeks or months to reach the target doses used in the large-scale trials.[81] In contrast to ACE inhibitors, for which it took more than 15 years of use before dose-ranging trials were completed,[82] the minimally effective dose is known for at least one β-blocker, carvedilol. Although the dose-ranging study with carvedilol supports increasing the dose to 25 mg bid, most of the relevant end points were significantly improved even at the lowest dose studied, 6.25 mg bid.[83] Although tempting to conclude that any dose of any hemodynamically active β-blocker would be acceptable, this may not

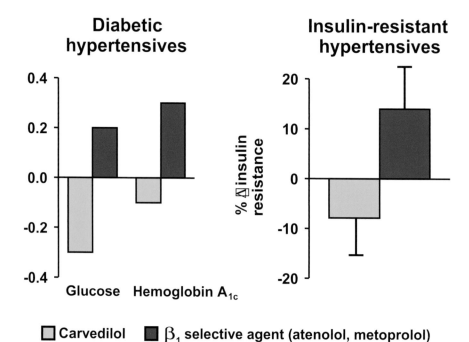

Figure 6. Different β-blockers have different effects on glucose metabolism. The results from small, short-term mechanistic studies suggesting that carvedilol would be a superior β-blocker for heart failure patients with diabetes or insulin resistance[70,71] parallel the report from the COMET trial that carvedilol therapy is associated with significantly less risk of developing diabetes than metoprolol tartrate therapy (Poole-Wilson P, presented at the annual meeting of the European Society of Cardiology, Vienna, Austria, August 30 to September 2, 2003). (From Sackner-Bernstein J, Kelly K. Before it happens to you: a breakthrough program for reversing or preventing heart disease. Cambridge, MA, Da Capo Press, 2004. Copyrighted by and used with permission from Jonathan Sackner-Bernstein, MD.)

be a safe conclusion to apply to β-blockers for which dose-ranging data are not available; thus, the lack of these data for metoprolol and bisoprolol could be a limitation. However, each of these drugs has been shown to be effective in clinical trials with a strategy of increasing the dose to the maximally tolerated one, and this should be the plan in clinical practice. On average, patients tolerate well the titration up to the target dose. During this initiation phase, sicker patients are at higher risk for developing fluid retention and symptomatic hypotension if the dose is escalated rapidly at weekly intervals,[84] but the risk of these side effects is not increased when the dose is increased more gradually; in fact, the risk of worsening heart failure is reduced within the first weeks of administration.[85] For most patients, this risk is not a major problem, and management of these side effects is generally successful when the rate of dose escalation is slowed and background therapies are adjusted.[81] In fact, β-blockers can be administered safely to patients with symptoms at rest or with minimal exertion, as demonstrated in the Carvedilol Prospective Randomized Cumulative Survival Study Group (COPERNICUS) trial.[16]

ACE Inhibitors

Clinical Trials

ACE inhibitors are proven therapy for patients with ventricular dysfunction, whether symptomatic or not (Fig. 7).[6-8,10,12,13] Recent studies have supported the use of ACE inhibitors in limiting the initial myocardial injury that leads to heart failure, both in acute myocardial infarction[9,86-88] and for patients at risk for developing heart failure.[12] The Heart Outcomes Prevention Evaluation (HOPE) study provided compelling data to

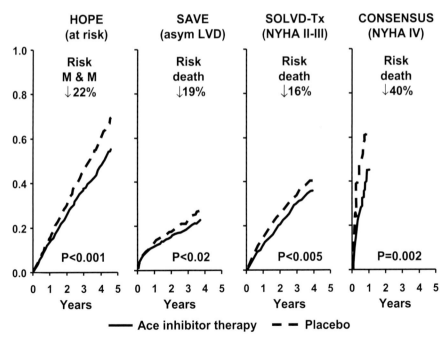

Figure 7. Angiotensin-converting enzyme (ACE) inhibitors reduce risk for patients with stage A heart failure and those with symptomatic disease.[6,7,10,12] Asym, asymptomatic; LVD, left ventricular dysfunction; M & M, morbidity and mortality; NYHA, New York Heart Association. (From Sackner-Bernstein J, Kelly K. Before it happens to you: a breakthrough program for reversing or preventing heart disease. Cambridge, MA, Da Capo Press, 2004. Copyrighted by and used with permission from Jonathan Sackner-Bernstein, MD.)

use ACE inhibitors more widely. The trial assessed the role of the ACE inhibitor ramipril on cardiovascular events, survival, and the development of heart failure in 9,533 patients. The population studied did not meet the "standard" criteria for ACE inhibitor therapy: their blood pressure was controlled and ventricular function was normal, but they were at high risk for cardiac events (they had either vascular disease or diabetes with at least one other coronary risk factor). The primary end point of cardiovascular death and major morbidity was reduced by 22% and the risk of heart failure by 23%.[12] EUROPA studied the effects of the ACE inhibitor perindopril on patients with previously diagnosed coronary heart disease. The study demonstrated a 20% reduction in the risk of cardiovascular death, myocardial infarction, or cardiac arrest.[13] These data mandate that ACE inhibitors become first-line therapy for patients with vascular disease, including those with cerebrovascular or coronary artery disease, in addition to those with the traditional coronary risk factors.

Drug Selection

The debate about the potential superiority of some agents over others focuses on pharmacokinetic and pharmacodynamic differences because there are no comparative studies with outcome data. Agents with longer half-lives would appear to afford a dosing advantage, resulting in better patient compliance. Other agents have a greater distribution into tissues, potentially affecting the local renin-angiotensin-aldosterone system (RAAS) in the vascular endothelium and myocardium. In a comparative study, a tissue-binding ACE inhibitor had a significantly greater effect on peripheral arterial vasodilation than a nonbinding agent.[89] However, no study has considered the clinical effect of this pharmacologic property, although the tissue-binding properties of an ACE inhibitor can be important.

Two lines of evidence suggest advantages of tissue avidity. In sudden death and acute myocardial infarction, plaque rupture is the pathoanatomical trigger. Studies have shown that angiotensin II and activated immune cells colocalize to the site of rupture[90] and increase the activation of the metalloproteinases that lead to plaque rupture.[91] Therefore, if one agent could penetrate into the tissue and interrupt the production of angiotensin II, it could be clinically beneficial. Importantly, such a benefit has not been demonstrated and is not being considered in any ongoing trial. However, the possibility of benefit cannot be ignored. An additional advantage for a tissue-avid ACE inhibitor is related to the frequency of administration. For example, ramiprilat, the active form of ramipril, has a half-life of only 2 to 4 hours. This would suggest the need for dosing three times daily; however, ramiprilat has triphasic elimination kinetics, that is, ramiprilat is absorbed into the plasma, rapidly distributed to the tissues, and then released from the tissues back into the circulation. This results in an effective half-life of more than 50 hours.[92] Therefore, even without clinical outcome data, the tissue avidity of an ACE inhibitor can be an important factor in drug selection. Agents that bind to the tissues in this fashion can have an effective half-life long enough to be administered once daily, as would be the case for a non–tissue-avid agent with a much longer half-life, such as lisinopril. However, agents with a longer half-life may be less likely to cause dizziness and hypotension because of the gradual onset of action and more constant hemodynamic effects over the course of the day. Either strategy permits once-daily dosing, which would improve patient compliance. After an agent has been chosen, the target dose is generally the maximum tolerated. However, no general rule can be applied to all patients to determine when the maximum tolerated dose has been achieved, especially when blood pressure starts to decrease or functional azotemia develops. The standard recommendation has been to use the doses shown by randomized clinical trials to be effective.[2]

Recently, two large studies compared the clinical effects of low-dose and high-dose ACE inhibitor therapy. The NETWORK study evaluated the effects of enalapril, 2.5, 5, and 10 mg bid, over 6 months in 1,500 patients with chronic heart failure. The study did not demonstrate any difference between the doses used in relation to all-cause mortality.[93] The Assessment of Treatment with Lisinopril and Survival (ATLAS)[82] study enrolled 3,164 patients (followed for a mean of 3.5 years) and compared 2.5-5 mg daily of lisinopril with 32.5-35 mg daily. Although ATLAS did not demonstrate a difference in its primary end point, all-cause mortality, the 12% decrease in the combined end point of death and hospitalization supports the use of higher doses when tolerated. Perhaps of most interest, patients taking a high dose of lisinopril tolerated the drug well and had a lower incidence of cough,[82] likely because improved cardiac filling pressures with higher doses reduce the frequency of cough caused by pulmonary hypertension and congestion. This indicates that any patient who experiences cough while taking an ACE inhibitor should have the dose increased as aggressively as possible to determine whether the patient can tolerate ACE inhibition and realize its clinical benefits. If this strategy is not effective, the dose of diuretics can be increased. Doubling the dose once or even for several days can be sufficient to reduce subclinical congestion, and if body weight decreases and the cough does not improve, it becomes more likely that the cough is ACE inhibitor-induced. Importantly, cough is common in patients with heart failure, but a review of clinical trials of ACE inhibitors has shown that the placebo group experienced cough almost as frequently as the ACE inhibitor group.[7,10] Although the results of the ATLAS study can be interpreted as evidence to treat patients with low doses of ACE inhibitors, many patients feel better with higher doses. Clinical practice should follow the strategy of the large-scale, randomized, placebo-controlled trials that proved the effectiveness of ACE inhibitors, that is, titrate the dose over several weeks to the maximum tolerated. This will provide the maximum benefit of neurohormonal blockade.

Metabolic Effects
ACE inhibitors are also useful for correcting metabolic abnormalities in heart failure. Insulin resistance improves with ACE inhibitors,[94-96] which is especially

important in heart failure because of the tendency for diuretics to make it worse.[95-97] This corrective effect occurs independently of angiotensin II activity and may represent an advantage of ACE inhibitors over angiotensin receptor blockers.[94,98] Also, ACE inhibitors reduce proteinuria[99] and slow the progression to renal failure in hypertension, a common comorbid condition in heart failure. Recent trials with the angiotensin receptor blockers losartan[100] and irbesartan[101] demonstrated similar effects in patients with type 2 diabetes, indicating that the mechanism is related largely to antagonism of angiotensin II.

Strategies for Clinical Practice

Treatment guidelines for the use of ACE inhibitors in clinical practice describe starting doses, target doses, and side effects.[1,2] Two factors that often lead to inappropriate drug withdrawal deserve particular attention. First, modest azotemia does not necessarily indicate impending renal failure or the presence of clinically significant renal artery stenosis. Because angiotensin II vasoconstricts the efferent arteriole of the glomerulus, a decrease in the amount of angiotensin II produced through ACE inhibition or angiotensin receptor blockade should decrease the filtration force within the glomerulus, leading to "functional" azotemia.[102]   In this case, a slight increase in the level of creatinine of 0.2 to 0.5 mg/dL should be accepted if it remains stable, although the level of tolerance becomes less for patients with a baseline creatinine above 2.0 mg/dL and even less if the baseline is above 2.5 mg/dL. If the creatinine level becomes markedly increased, the diagnosis of renal artery stenosis should be pursued. Second, lack of a therapeutic benefit after only a few days or weeks should not lead to drug withdrawal because these agents produce short-term effects that may vary greatly from long-term effects,[103] and they may not produce clinically measurable effects for up to 3 months.[104] Furthermore, these agents can prevent progression of disease and reduce the risk of death, even in the absence of improved quality of life.[10] Patients who are more likely to experience side effects early in treatment can be identified, for example, sicker patients with hyponatremia[105] or patients with diabetes,[106] marked renal dysfunction,[107] or marked activation of the RAAS, including those who have recently had a large-volume diuresis. Patients who have low right atrial pressure ($\leq$12 mm Hg) and preserved renal function (creatinine, <1.5 mg/dL) appear twice as likely to have clinical improvement than those with high right atrial pressure and an abnormal creatinine level.[108]

Angiotensin Receptor Antagonists

Rationale

In contrast to ACE inhibitor therapy, which prevents the adverse effects of angiotensin II by blocking its synthesis through ACE, angiotensin receptor blockers prevent angiotensin II from acting on the cell by selectively blocking angiotensin II type 1 (AT_1) receptors. This prevents vasoconstriction, sodium retention, hypertrophy, and fibrosis. Also, the effects of angiotensin II as a positive inotrope and a stimulus for the secretion of endothelin and the release of norepinephrine are blocked.[109] Angiotensin receptor blockade effectively treats hypertension and improves cardiac filling pressures in patients with heart failure.[110,111] Because angiotensin II can be produced by enzymatic pathways in addition to the ACE pathway,[109] the level of angiotensin II begins to increase months or years after therapy is initiated with an ACE inhibitor.[112,113] Therefore, angiotensin receptor blockers may be a more direct way to block the effects of activation of the RAAS in heart failure.

Clinical Trials

Initially, angiotensin receptor blockers were evaluated as an alternative to ACE inhibitors for patients with heart failure because they were expected to be as effective as ACE inhibitors but with less azotemia and a lower incidence of cough. Although the hemodynamic effects were similar to those of ACE inhibitors, the Evaluation of Losartan in the Elderly (ELITE I) trial was the first study to consider the clinical effect of these agents. The results of this study appeared to show a reduction in the risk of sudden death with losartan compared with captopril, but the study was not definitive because this analysis was a secondary end point for which the statistical power was not robust.[114] A second trial, ELITE II, attempted to confirm the observation, but the results appeared to favor the ACE inhibitor, although the differences did not reach statistical significance.[115] The investigators concluded that of the two classes, ACE inhibitors are the therapy of choice. In the Randomized Evaluation of Strategies for Left Ventricular Dysfunction (RESOLVD) study, candesartan was evaluated in comparison with enalapril and the combination of candesartan and enalapril. This study was not designed to assess the effect on clinical end points but rather on neurohormonal activation and left ventricular remodeling. However, patients in the angiotensin receptor blocker group did not appear to respond as well as those in the enalapril alone group, although there were no significant differences.[116] These trials did not consider the equally important issue of whether angiotensin receptor blockers are useful when added to ACE inhibitor therapy.

Two trials were designed to assess the safety and efficacy of combined ACE inhibitor and angiotensin receptor blocker therapy in chronic heart failure: the Valsartan Heart Failure Trial (Val-HeFT)[59] and CHARM trial.[60] The results of Val-HeFT support the use of valsartan for treating chronic heart failure in patients who are intolerant of ACE inhibitors (44% reduction in the combined risk of death or hospitalization), but the study raised questions about the addition of this agent to the treatment of patients already receiving ACE inhibitors and β-blockers. For these patients, the addition of valsartan was associated with a trend toward increased risk of death or hospitalization (RR=1.18, P=NS) and toward a higher risk of death (RR=1.41, P=NS).[59] These estimates cannot be considered definitive because of the nature of subgroup analyses and the level of statistical significance, even though randomization was stratified to the use of β-blockers. These trends were strong enough to warrant restraint when considering combination therapy with β-blockers, ACE inhibitors, and angiotensin receptor blockers.

Strategies for Clinical Practice

Before the results of CHARM were available, angiotensin receptor blockers were prescribed for heart failure patients intolerant of ACE inhibitors or who had side effects deemed untenable. Because none of these agents had been shown to improve clinical outcomes in addition to ACE inhibition and β-blockade, no angiotensin receptor blocker was considered standard therapy in the treatment of heart failure except in the case of tolerance of ACE inhibitors. However, the results of CHARM are sufficiently relevant clinically (not merely statistically) that candesartan should be standard treatment for patients with heart failure who remain symptomatic despite ACE inhibitor and β-blocker therapy in a volume-optimized patient. There are insufficient data to generalize the strategy to the entire class of angiotensin receptor blockers (Fig. 8).

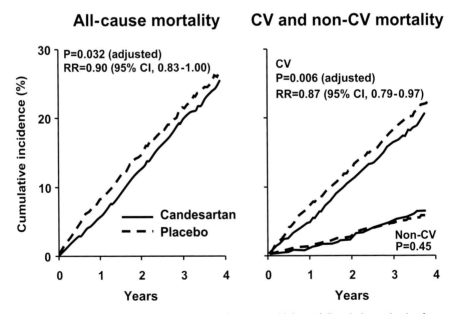

Figure 8. Candesartan improves outcomes of patients with heart failure independently of level of ventricular dysfunction. (From Pfeffer et al.[60] By permission of Elsevier.)

Aldosterone Antagonists

Activation of the RAAS leads to progression of heart failure through the effects of angiotensin II as well as aldosterone. The effects of aldosterone are similar to those of angiotensin II, especially in relation to volume expansion and myocardial fibrosis.[117] Its contribution to disease progression was confirmed by the beneficial effects of anti-aldosterone therapy with spironolactone in patients with advanced heart failure.[20] In this study, patients with recent class IV symptoms who were still affected by NYHA class III-IV symptoms after optimal therapy were treated with spironolactone or placebo. Spironolactone significantly reduced the risk of death in this population. Eplerenone was recently approved by the U.S. Food and Drug Administration (FDA) for the treatment of hypertension and to reduce the risk of death (and major morbidity) in patients with left ventricular dysfunction and heart failure symptoms after myocardial infarction, that is, those with stage B or C heart failure (Fig. 9).[21]

Strategies for Clinical Practice

Aldosterone antagonists are proven to reduce risk in patients with advanced heart failure and those with left ventricular dysfunction and heart failure symptoms after

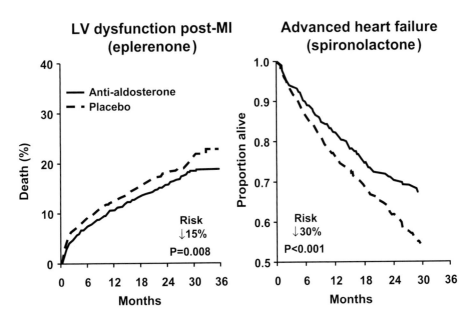

Figure 9. Anti-aldosterone therapy reduces risk for patients with left ventricular (LV) dysfunction post-myocardial infarction (MI) and for those with advanced heart failure. (From Pitt et al.[20,21] By permission of the Massachusetts Medical Society.)

myocardial infarction. Although the studies are not as numerous as for ACE inhibitors or β-blockers, the results of the two primary trials are concordant and apply to patients at the two extremes of the disease process, that is, early after infarction and advanced chronic heart failure. From the available data, it is not possible to identify patients who may be at higher risk for hyperkalemia. Therefore, monitoring potassium levels closely is crucial, especially in patients with increased creatinine levels (>2.0 mg/dL) or a history of hyperkalemia. In addition, during hot months or at other times when patients may be prone to even mild dehydration, close observation would appear prudent.

Summary

Compelling clinical trial data mandate that all patients with heart failure receive treatment with ACE inhibitors and β-blockers. In addition, recent data support more widespread use of anti-aldosterone therapy as well as the use of angiotensin receptor antagonism (particularly candesartan). Therefore, the first step to optimize treatment of heart failure is to prescribe ACE inhibitors and β-blockers for all patients who could experience benefit. Without doubt, the use of these agents should begin at the time of acute myocardial infarction and treatment with them should be started in any patient who has ventricular dysfunction and does not have volume overload or an unstable condition. The HOPE and EUROPA[118] studies proved that ACE inhibitors should also be administered to patients at risk for cardiovascular events.[12] Although no study has addressed this issue directly, β-blockers also would appear to be rational therapy for patients at risk, considering the pathophysiology of hypertension, coronary artery disease, and heart failure. In accordance with this view, the recent AHA/ACC guidelines recommend that diabetic, hypertensive, and hypercholesterolemic patients in stage A heart failure should be treated with medications that are also safe and effective for stages B, C, and D. This recommendation means that ACE inhibitors and β-blockers should be used as first-line therapy, particularly for patients with hypertension or coronary artery disease. Although some may argue that this contradicts the recommendations of stepped therapy in the Seventh Report of the Joint National Committee on Detection, Evaluation, and Treatment of High Blood Pressure (JNC-VII), it is in fact a more rational approach.

Consider a typical 50-year-old patient. Recent studies with intravascular ultrasonography suggest that the likelihood of clinically significant coronary atherosclerosis for this patient is at least 75%.[119] With such a high likelihood of disease on the basis of age or by applying the Framingham risk calculation, this patient is best managed as if he or she already has coronary artery disease. In fact, the medications for preventing cardiac events are the same ones that can control blood pressure: ACE inhibitors and β-blockers. Therefore, the optimal strategy should not stop with widespread use of ACE inhibitors and β-blockers for patients with symptomatic heart failure but should be extended to include treatment of patients at risk for developing heart failure. This is a patient with stage A disease, that is, a patient with hypertension, coronary artery disease, hypercholesterolemia, or diabetes or a combination of these.

Practical Approach

The most rapid and reliable way to improve the symptoms of patients with congestive heart failure is through the judicious use of diuretics. Importantly, patients who have volume overload are not optimal candidates for starting treatment with β-blockers or ACE inhibitors until their volume status has been optimized. When β-blocker therapy is initiated with rapidly increasing doses, the risk of worsening fluid retention is high.[84] In contrast, even patients with advanced heart failure tolerate the initiation of β-blocker therapy if low starting doses are gradually increased no more frequently than every 2 weeks.[85] Recent data indicate that β-blocker therapy can be initiated at the time of hospitalization, after a patient's condition has been stabilized, before discharge.[120] Patients with volume overload and increased right atrial pressure have a response rate to ACE inhibitor therapy of less than 50%,[108] but these agents can be introduced safely and effectively in a patient whose condition has been stabilized.

The findings of the CHARM study support an important role for the angiotensin receptor blocker candesartan. Before CHARM, these agents had not been proved beneficial in the studies that had been completed except for patients who are intolerant of ACE inhibitors. In contrast, aldosterone antagonism is useful for patients with advanced disease and those with ventricular dysfunction after myocardial infarction,[21] but its use requires close monitoring of potassium concentrations for several weeks, especially when given in conjunction with β-blockade and high-dose ACE inhibition.

In clinical practice, the following algorithm should be followed. First, use diuretics to rid the patient of excess volume. This will permit the safe and effective introduction of β-blocker and ACE inhibitor therapy. ACE inhibitors can be introduced and increased over the course of 1 to 2 weeks except in the sickest patients, who will require a more gradual schedule. For the first 2 weeks after initiation of treatment, renal function and electrolytes should be monitored (more frequently in sicker patients and in those with baseline creatinine concentrations above 1.5 mg/dL). After the optimal dose has been established and renal function is stable, the β-blocker dose can be increased. This titration should be more gradual, and patients should be evaluated at each increment in dose. Persistent dizziness can be treated with a temporary reduction in the dose of ACE inhibitor or diuretic, depending on the clinical scenario, and fluid retention responds to an increased diuretic dose that generally permits a continued but more gradual up-titration. In patients with ventricular dysfunction after myocardial infarction[21] and those with chronic heart failure,[20] anti-aldosterone therapy is indicated. Those with symptomatic heart failure despite maximum therapy should receive an angiotensin receptor blocker, as shown in CHARM, independently of the ejection fraction.[60]

Clinical effects of neurohormonal antagonism include improvement in functional status and ventricular function, but even in the absence of such changes, these agents reduce the risk of disease progression and death. These are the ultimate targets of optimal neurohormonal antagonism in patients with heart failure and ventricular dysfunction and can be achieved by widespread use of β-blockers and ACE inhibitors. Available data mandate ACE inhibitor therapy for patients at risk for developing heart failure.[12] Also, the clinical practice of using β-blockers earlier in the development of heart failure appears rational.

Aggressive Treatment of Patients With Stage A Heart Failure

The AHA/ACC heart failure guidelines define stage A heart failure to include patients with hypertension, dyslipidemia, coronary artery disease, or diabetes. Their management is reviewed briefly below.

Hypertension

JNC-7 advocates the treatment of hypertension to a goal of less than 140/90 mm Hg.[121] However, the guidelines cite evidence that indicates risk is minimized when a pressure of 115/75 mm Hg is achieved (Fig. 10 and 11).[122] The reason for this disparity is not clear from the information published by the committee. The major reason is likely the cost to society of such an aggressive strategy, with additional concern based on the lack of a randomized, controlled trial to prove that further lowering of blood pressure is warranted. In the setting of left ventricular dysfunction, minimizing hemodynamic load appears justified, and the lower blood pressure target should be preferred for patients with ventricular dysfunction, if not the population in general.

The HOPE trial considered the issue of treating "borderline" hypertension. In this trial, systolic blood pressure was in the mid 130s[12] and, based on ambulatory blood pressure measurements in a subset of patients, was reduced by 10/4 mm Hg.[123] This effect occurred in parallel with a reduction in vascular events of 22%,[12] supporting the usefulness of more aggressive control of blood pressure.

Dyslipidemia

Similarly, the report of the National Cholesterol Education Panel Adult Treatment Program[124] has set targets that are not associated with the lowest possible risk. This document explicitly states that the barrier to more aggressive treatment is its cost-effectiveness and argues that when statins cost less than $500 per year, the recommendations should be more aggressive. On the basis of the data reviewed in the report, it appears likely that optimal treatment would be

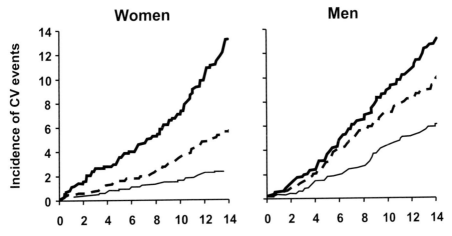

Population	Women	Men
▬ High-normal (130-139/95-89)	891	903
▬ ▬ Normal (120-129/80-84)	1,126	1,059
▬ Optimal (<120/80)	1,875	1,005

Figure 10. The Seventh Report of the Joint National Committee on Prevention, Detection, Evaluation, and Treatment of High Blood Pressure targets of 140/90 mm Hg do not minimize risk. CV, cardiovascular. (From Vasan RS, Larson MG, Leip EP, Evans JC, O'Donnell CJ, Kannel WB, et al. Impact of high-normal blood pressure on the risk of cardiovascular disease. N Engl J Med 2001;345:1291-7. By permission of the Massachusetts Medical Society.)

achieved when low-density lipoprotein (LDL)-cholesterol is reduced below 100 mg/dL and possibly lower if there is clinically significant coronary artery disease.

The Heart Protection Study demonstrated that simvastatin markedly reduces risk even when the LDL and total cholesterol levels appear sufficiently low (Fig. 12). For diabetic patients with a total cholesterol of at least 135 mg/dL, 40 mg of simvastatin nightly significantly reduced the risk of vascular events.[125] Independently of the presence of diabetes, the use of statins for hypercholesterolemia in patients with ischemic cardiomyopathy, whether as a primary or secondary prevention strategy, reduces the risks of death, myocardial infarction, and stroke.[29-31,125] Probably because of the reduced risk of myocardial infarction, statins also reduce the risk of overt heart failure.[32] Although patients with end-stage heart failure can be cachectic and have hypocholesterolemia, the patients commonly seen in practice are ambulatory and unlikely to have such metabolic disarray.

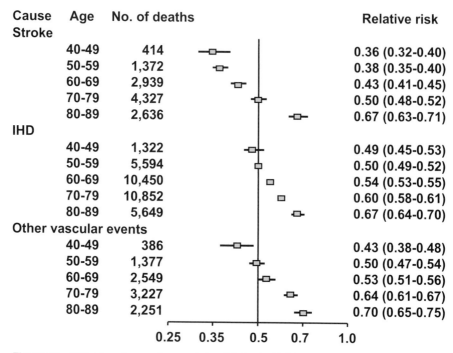

Figure 11. Risk of cardiovascular events is minimized with blood pressure of 115/75 mm Hg (or at least a 20 mm Hg decrease). IHD, ischemic heart disease. (From Lewington et al.[122] By permission of Elsevier.)

Coronary Artery Disease

Many patients have heart failure and ischemic heart disease and are treated long-term with a low dose of aspirin. Although some may criticize this strategy because of the possibility of an adverse interaction between aspirin and ACE inhibitors[126] as well as the recently reported suggestion of an interaction between aspirin and β-blocker therapy,[118] the standard practice is to treat patients with coronary heart disease with long-term aspirin therapy. The studies that suggested an adverse interaction do not report a negative effect, only an attenuation of the benefit of the ACE inhibitor or β-blocker. However, these reports discount the beneficial effect of aspirin therapy in those for whom it is indicated.

Diabetes Mellitus

Several trials have established that the risk of cardiovascular events and end-organ damage are reduced with optimal glucose control.[127] Less commonly known is the

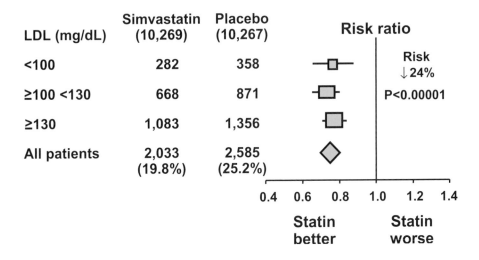

Figure 12. Heart Protection Study: the risk of clinical events is reduced in patients with vascular disease, even with low LDL. (From MRC/BHF Heart Protection Study: HPS Info—Slideshow Presentation. Available at: http://www.ctsu.ox.ac.uk/~hps/hps_slides.shtml. Accessed October 23, 2003. By permission of the British Heart Foundation.)

extent of undiagnosed diabetes. Although the disease affects almost 2.5% of the American population, some estimate that twice as many have undiagnosed diabetes.[128] Diabetic men have twice the risk of developing heart failure and diabetic women five times the risk,[39] forcing us to address diabetes management to reduce the burden of heart failure. Likely, millions more of the population are insulin-resistant. The state of insulin resistance is not very different from the state of asymptomatic ventricular dysfunction. In both cases, these states are steps between "normal" and a diseased state. In either case, introduction of therapy earlier in the process is rational, even if it is not an FDA-approved approach. After all, the goal is to prevent progression of disease. If a therapy can safely prevent progression, it should be introduced in this early stage. For heart failure, ACE inhibitor and β-blocker therapy can be introduced safely; however, for insulin resistance, we lack a proven therapeutic strategy to prevent diabetes in patients with heart failure who are insulin-resistant,[129] because metformin is relatively contraindicated in the presence of heart failure. Nonetheless, screening for subclinical diabetes by measuring fasting glucose and glycohemoglobin levels should be standard practice for patients with heart failure, because of reports of insulin resistance in these patients.[78] Dietary counseling and an evaluation for reversible causes of glucose intolerance should follow for appropriate patients. An example of a simple issue to consider is a patient taking a β_1-selective β-blocker. In both diabetic and nondiabetic patients with hypertension, metoprolol[70] and atenolol[71] have been shown to worsen insulin resistance compared with the combined β-α-blocker carvedilol. Therefore, mild increases in glycohemoglobin in patients receiving selective β-blockers indicate that treatment should be switched to carvedilol and the glycohemoglobin concentration measured again in 2 or 3 months. Without doubt, all diabetic patients should be treated with an ACE inhibitor[12] unless there is a specific contraindication, and statin therapy is indicated irrespective of cholesterol level (as long as total cholesterol is above 135 mg/dL, the entry criteria for the Heart Protection Study).[125,130]

Conclusions

Investigators and pharmaceutical companies have focused on the next neurohormonal antagonist, one to complement β-blockers, ACE inhibitors, and angiotensin receptor antagonists, but have failed. The nature of investigators is to search for the new target and the new therapy in an attempt to change the natural history of disease. Yet, the data indicate that the breakthrough treatment for heart failure—and for those at risk for developing it—already exists. Only a fraction of eligible patients are treated with optimized doses of β-blockers, ACE inhibitors, angiotensin receptor blockers, or aldosterone antagonists. The challenge is to apply the principles of evidence-based medicine and to translate research findings into clinical practice. Treating stages A, B, C, and D heart failure with β-blockers and ACE inhibitors is the optimal strategy for neurohormonal antagonism, and concentrating particularly on patients with early disease will have the greatest effect possible on the natural history of the disease.

When disease progresses despite these therapies, biventricular pacing improves quality of life for those with underlying dyssynchronous ventricular contraction. The risk of sudden death for patients with ischemic cardiomyopathy is markedly reduced by defibrillators, and in all likelihood, ongoing trials will initially broaden the population of candidates for these devices, and subsequent understanding of the underlying cellular and molecular mechanisms will permit more precise and targeted patient selection.

References

1. Packer M, Cohn JN, editors. Consensus recommendations for the management of chronic heart failure. Am J Cardiol 1999;83 Suppl 2A:1A-38A.

2. Guideline Committee Members and the Executive Council for the Heart Failure Society of America. HFSA guidelines for management of patients with heart failure caused by left ventricular systolic dysfunction: pharmacological approaches [published erratum appears in J Card Fail 2000;6:74]. J Card Fail 1999;5:357-82.

3. Hunt SA, Baker DW, Chin MH, Cinquegrani MP, Feldman AM, Francis GS, et al. ACC/AHA guidelines for the evaluation and management of chronic heart failure in the adult: executive summary. A report of the American College of Cardiology/American Heart Association Task Force on Practice Guidelines (Committee to Revise the 1995 Guidelines for the Evaluation and Management of Heart Failure). Circulation 2001:104:2996-3007.

4. Remme WJ, Swedberg K, Task Force for the Diagnosis and Treatment of Chronic Heart Failure, European Society of Cardiology. Guidelines for the diagnosis and treatment of chronic heart failure [published erratum appears in Eur Heart J 2001;22:2217-8]. Eur Heart J 2001;22:1527-60.

5. Jessup M, Brozena S. Heart failure. N Engl J Med 2003:348:2007-18.

6. The CONSENSUS Trial Study Group. Effects of enalapril on mortality in severe congestive heart failure: results of the Cooperative North Scandinavian Enalapril Survival Study (CONSENSUS). N Engl J Med 1987;316:1429-35.

7. The SOLVD Investigators. Effect of enalapril on survival in patients with reduced left ventricular ejection fractions and congestive heart failure. N Engl J Med 1991;325:293-302.

8. The SOLVD Investigators. Effect of enalapril on mortality and the development of heart failure in asymptomatic patients with reduced left ventricular ejection fractions [published erratum appears in N Engl J Med 1992;327:1768]. N Engl J Med 1992;327:685-91.

9. The Acute Infarction Ramipril Efficacy (AIRE) Study Investigators. Effect of ramipril on mortality and morbidity of survivors of acute myocardial infarction with clinical evidence of heart failure. Lancet 1993;342:821-8.

10. Pfeffer MA, Braunwald E, Moye LA, Basta L, Brown EJ Jr, Cuddy TE, et al., the SAVE Investigators. Effect of captopril on mortality and morbidity in patients with left ventricular dysfunction after myocardial infarction: results of the survival and ventricular enlargement trial. N Engl J Med 1992;327:669-77.

11. Torp-Pedersen C, Kober L, Carlsen J. Angio-converting enzyme inhibition after myocardial infarction: the Trandolapril Cardiac Evaluation Study. Am Heart J 1996;132:235-43.

12. The Heart Outcomes Prevention Evaluation Study Investigators. Effects of an angiotensin-converting-enzyme inhibitor, ramipril, on cardiovascular events in high-risk patients [published errata appear in N Engl J Med 2000;342:748, 2000;342:1376]. N Engl J Med 2000;342:145-53.

13. The EURopean trial On reduction of cardiac events with Perindopril in stable coronary Artery disease Investigators. Efficacy of perindopril in reduction of cardiovascular events among patients with stable coronary artery disease: randomised, double-blind, placebo-controlled, multicentre trial (the EUROPA study). Lancet 2003;362:782-8.

14. The Cardiac Insufficiency Bisoprolol Study II (CIBIS-II): a randomised trial. Lancet 1999;353:9-13.

15. Effect of metoprolol CR/XL in chronic heart failure: Metoprolol CR/XL Randomised Intervention Trial in Congestive Heart Failure. Lancet 1999;353:2001-7.

16. Packer M, Coats AJ, Fowler MB, Katus HA, Krum H, Mohacsi P, et al., for the Carvedilol Prospective Randomized Cumulative Survival Study Group. Effect of carvedilol on survival in severe chronic heart failure. N Engl J Med 2001;344:1651-8.

17. Poole-Wilson PA, Swedberg K, Cleland JG, Di Lenarda A, Hanrath P, Komajda M, et al., and COMET Investigators. Comparison of carvedilol and metoprolol on clinical outcomes in patients with chronic heart failure in the Carvedilol Or Metoprolol European Trial (COMET): randomised controlled trial. Lancet 2003;362:7-13.

18. A randomized trial of propranolol in patients with acute myocardial infarction: II. morbidity results. JAMA 1983;250:2814-9.

19. Packer M, Bristow MR, Cohn JN, Colucci WS, Fowler MB, Gilbert EM, et al., for the U.S. Carvedilol Heart Failure Study Group. The effect of carvedilol on morbidity and mortality in patients with chronic heart failure. N Engl J Med 1996;334:1349-55.

20. Pitt B, Zannad F, Remme WJ, Cody R, Castaigne A, Perez A, et al., for the Randomized Aldactone Evaluation Study Investigators. The effect of spironolactone on morbidity and mortality in patients with severe heart failure. N Engl J Med 1999;341:709-17.

21. Pitt B, Remme W, Zannad F, Neaton J, Martinez F, Roniker B, et al., for the Eplerenone Post-Acute Myocardial Infarction Heart Failure Efficacy and Survival Study Investigators. Eplerenone, a selective aldosterone blocker, in patients with left ventricular dysfunction after myocardial infarction [published erratum appears in N Engl J Med 2003;348:2271]. N Engl J Med 2003;348:1309-21.

22. Moss AJ, Hall WJ, Cannom DS, Daubert JP, Higgins SL, Klein H, et al., for the Multicenter Automatic Defibrillator Implantation Trial Investigators. Improved survival with an implanted defibrillator in patients with coronary disease at high risk for ventricular arrhythmia. N Engl J Med 1996;335:1933-40.

23. Rose EA, Gelijns AC, Moskowitz AJ, Heitjan DF, Stevenson LW, Dembitsky W, et al., for the Randomized Evaluation of Mechanical Assistance for the Treatment of Congestive Heart Failure (REMATCH) Study Group. Long-term mechanical left ventricular assistance for end-stage heart failure. N Engl J Med 2001;345:1435-43.

24. Abraham WT, Fisher WG, Smith AL, Delurgio DB, Leon AR, Loh E, et al., for the MIRACLE Study Group. Cardiac resynchronization in chronic heart failure. N Engl J Med 2002;346:1845-53.

25. Moss AJ, Zareba W, Hall WJ, Klein H, Wilber DJ, Cannom DS, et al., for the Multicenter Automatic Defibrillator Implantation Trial II Investigators. Prophylactic implantation of a defibrillator in patients with myocardial infarction and reduced ejection fraction. N Engl J Med 2002;346:877-83.

26. Young JB, Abraham WT, Smith AL, Leon AR, Lieberman R, Wilkoff B, Canby RC, et al., for the Multicenter InSync ICD Randomized Clinical Evaluation (MIRACLE ICD) Trial Investigators. Combined cardiac resynchronization and implantable cardioversion defibrillation in advanced chronic heart failure: the MIRACLE ICD Trial. JAMA 2003;289:2685-94.

27. The Digitalis Investigation Group. The effect of digoxin on mortality and morbidity in patients with heart failure. N Engl J Med 1997;336:525-33.

28. Cohn JN. The management of chronic heart failure. N Engl J Med 1996;335:490-8.

29. Randomised trial of cholesterol lowering in 4444 patients with coronary heart disease: the Scandinavian Simvastatin Survival Study (4S). Lancet 1994;344:1383-9.

30. Sacks FM, Pfeffer MA, Moye LA, Rouleau JL, Rutherford JD, Cole TG, et al, for the Cholesterol and Recurrent Events Trial Investigators. The effect of pravastatin on coronary events after myocardial infarction in patients with average cholesterol levels. N Engl J Med 1996;335:1001-9.

31. The Long-Term Intervention with Pravastatin in Ischaemic Disease (LIPID) Study Group. Prevention of cardiovascular events and death with pravastatin in patients with coronary heart disease and a broad range of initial cholesterol levels. N Engl J Med 1998;339:1349-57.

32. Kjekshus J, Pedersen TR, Olsson AG, Faergeman O, Pyorala K. The effects of simvastatin on the incidence of heart failure in patients with coronary heart disease [published erratum appears in J Card Fail 1998;4:367]. J Card Fail 1997;3:249-54.

33. Bristow MR, Saxon LA, Boehmer J, Krueger S, McGrew F, Botteron G, et al., for the COMPANION Investigators. Cardiac resynchronization therapy (CRT) reduces hospitalizations, and CRT + an implantable defibrillator (CRT-D) reduces mortality in chronic heart failure: preliminary results of the COMPANION trial. Retrieved August 29, 2003, from the World Wide Web: http://www.uchsc.edu/cvi/clb.pdf.

34. Davies M, Hobbs F, Davis R, Kenkre J, Roalfe AK, Hare R, et al. Prevalence of left-ventricular systolic dysfunction and heart failure in the Echocardiographic Heart of England Screening study: a population based study. Lancet 2001;358:439-44.

35. American Heart Association. Heart Disease and Stroke Statistics—2003 Update. Dallas, TX: American Heart Association; 2002. Retrieved October 6, 2003 from the World Wide Web: http://www.americanheart.org/downloadable/heart/1040391091015HDS_Stats_03.pdf.

36. Mandel JS, Church TR, Bond JH, Ederer F, Geisser MS, Mongin SJ, et al. The effect of fecal occult-blood screening on the incidence of colorectal cancer. N Engl J Med 2000;343:1603-7.

37. Mandel JS, Bond JH, Church TR, Snover DC, Bradley GM, Schuman LM, et al., for the Minnesota Colon Cancer Control Study. Reducing mortality from colorectal cancer by screening for fecal occult blood [published erratum appears in N Engl J Med 1993;329:672]. N Engl J Med 1993;328:1365-71.

38. American Cancer Society. Cancer Facts & Figures 2003. Atlanta, GA: American Cancer Society; 2003. Retrieved October 6, 2003 from the World Wide Web: http://www.cancer.org/docroot/STT/content/STT_1x_Cancer_Facts__Figures_2003.asp.

39. Kannel WB, D'Agostino RB, Silbershatz H, Belanger AJ, Wilson PW, Levy D. Profile for estimating risk of heart failure. Arch Intern Med 1999;159:1197-204.

40. Lloyd-Jones DM, Larson MG, Leip EP, Beiser A, D'Agostino RB, Kannel WB, et al. Lifetime risk for developing congestive heart failure: the Framingham Heart Study. Circulation 2002;106:3068-72.

41. Wald NJ, Law MR. A strategy to reduce cardiovascular disease by more than 80% [published erratum appears in BMJ 2003;327:586]. BMJ 2003;326:1419.

42. Yamamoto K, Burnett JC Jr, Jougasaki M, Nishimura RA, Bailey KR, Saito Y, et al. Superiority of brain natriuretic peptide as a hormonal marker of ventricular systolic and diastolic dysfunction and ventricular hypertrophy. Hypertension 1996;28:988-94.

43. Dao Q, Krishnaswamy P, Kazanegra R, Harrison A, Amirnovin R, Lenert L, et al. Utility of B-type natriuretic peptide in the diagnosis of congestive heart failure in an urgent-care setting. J Am Coll Cardiol 2001;37:379-85.

44. Troughton RW, Frampton CM, Yandle TG, Espiner EA, Nicholls MG, Richards AM. Treatment of heart failure guided by plasma aminoterminal brain natriuretic peptide (N-BNP) concentrations. Lancet 2000;355:1126-30.

45. Levy D, Kenchaiah S, Larson MG, Benjamin EJ, Kupka MJ, Ho KK, et al. Long-term trends in the incidence of and survival with heart failure. N Engl J Med 2002;347:1397-402.

46. Dargie HJ. Effect of carvedilol on outcome after myocardial infarction in patients with left-ventricular dysfunction: the CAPRICORN randomised trial. Lancet 2001;357:1385-90.

47. Rich MW, Beckham V, Wittenberg C, Leven CL, Freedland KE, Carney RM. A multidisciplinary intervention to prevent the readmission of elderly patients with congestive heart failure. N Engl J Med 1995;333:1190-5.

48. Sackner-Bernstein J. Congestive heart failure. In: Curtis JR, Rubenfeld GD, editors. Managing death in the intensive care unit: the transition from cure to comfort. New York: Oxford University Press; 2001. p. 311-7.

49. Mann DL. Mechanisms and models in heart failure: a combinatorial approach. Circulation 1999;100:999-1008.

50. Sackner-Bernstein JD. The myocardial matrix and the development and progression of ventricular remodeling. Curr Cardiol Rep 2000;2:112-9.

51. Colucci WS. The effects of norepinephrine on myocardial biology: implications for the therapy of heart failure. Clin Cardiol 1998;21 Suppl 1:I20-4.

52. St John Sutton M, Pfeffer MA, Plappert T, Rouleau JL, Moye LA, Dagenais GR, et al. Quantitative two-dimensional echocardiographic measurements are major predictors of adverse cardiovascular events after acute myocardial infarction: the protective effects of captopril. Circulation 1994;89:68-75.

53. Kostuk WJ, Kazamias TM, Gander MP, Simon AL, Ross J Jr. Left ventricular size after acute myocardial infarction: serial changes and their prognostic significance. Circulation 1973;47:1174-9.

54. Migrino RQ, Young JB, Ellis SG, White HD, Lundergan CF, Miller DP, et al., for the Global Utilization of Streptokinase and t-PA for Occluded Coronary Arteries (GUSTO)-I Angiographic Investigators. End-systolic volume index at 90 to 180 minutes into reperfusion therapy for acute myocardial infarction is a strong predictor of early and late mortality. Circulation 1997;96:116-21.

55. Silver MA. Success with heart failure: help and hope for those with congestive heart failure. Cambridge (MA): Perseus; 2002.

56. Chinese Cardiac Study (CCS-1) Collaborative Group. Oral captopril versus placebo among 14,962 patients with suspected acute myocardial infarction: a multicenter, randomized, double-blind, placebo controlled clinical trial. Chin Med J (Engl) 1997;110:834-8.

57. Olsson G, Tuomilehto J, Berglund G, Elmfeldt D, Warnold I, Barber H, et al. Primary prevention of sudden cardiovascular death in hypertensive patients: mortality results from the MAPHY Study. Am J Hypertens 1991;4:151-8.

58. Cohn JN, Archibald DG, Ziesche S, Franciosa JA, Harston WE, Tristani FE, et al. Effect of vasodilator therapy on mortality in chronic congestive heart failure: results of a Veterans Administration Cooperative Study. N Engl J Med 1986;314:1547-52.

59. Cohn JN, Tognoni G, for the Valsartan Heart Failure Trial Investigators. A randomized trial of the angiotensin-receptor blocker valsartan in chronic heart failure. N Engl J Med 2001;345:1667-75.

60. Pfeffer MA, Swedberg K, Granger CB, Held P, McMurray JJ, Michelson EL, et al., for the CHARM Investigators and Committees. Effects of candesartan on mortality and morbidity in patients with chronic heart failure: the CHARM-Overall programme. Lancet 2003;362:759-66.

61. Goldstein S. Propranolol therapy in patients with acute myocardial infarction: the Beta-Blocker Heart Attack Trial. Circulation 1983;67 Suppl I:I53-7.

62. Jones CG, Cleland JGF. Meeting report—the LIDO, HOPE, MOXCON and WASH studies. Eur J Heart Fail 1999;1:425-31.

63. The Beta-Blocker Evaluation of Survival Trial Investigators. A trial of the beta-blocker bucindolol in patients with advanced chronic heart failure. N Engl J Med 2001;344:1659-67.

64. Zebrack JS, Munger MA, MacGregor JF, Stoddard GJ, Gilbert EM. Beta receptor selectivity of carvedilol versus metoprolol succinate: a dose ranging study [abstract]. Circulation 2002;106 Suppl 2:II-612.

65. Kukin ML, Kalman J, Charney RH, Levy DK, Buchholz-Varley C, Ocampo ON, et al. Prospective, randomized comparison of effect of long-term treatment with metoprolol or carvedilol on symptoms, exercise, ejection fraction, and oxidative stress in heart failure. Circulation 1999;99:2645-51.

66. Sanderson JE, Chan SK, Yip G, Yeung LY, Chan KW, Raymond K, et al. Beta-blockade in heart failure: a comparison of carvedilol with metoprolol. J Am Coll Cardiol 1999;34:1522-8.

67. Di Lenarda A, Sabbadini G, Salvatore L, Sinagra G, Mestroni L, Pinamonti B, et al., and The Heart-Muscle Disease Study Group. J Am Coll Cardiol 1999;33:1926-34.

68. Metra M, Giubbini R, Nodari S, Boldi E, Modena MG, Dei Cas L. Differential effects of β-blockers in patients with heart failure: a prospective, randomized, double-blind comparison of the long-term effects of metoprolol versus carvedilol. Circulation 2000;102:546-51.

69. Swedberg K, Bergh CH, Dickstein K, McNay J, Steinberg M, and Moxonidine Investigators. The effects of moxonidine, a novel imidazoline, on plasma norepinephrine in patients with congestive heart failure. J Am Coll Cardiol 2000;35:398-404.

70. Jacob S, Rett K, Wicklmayr M, Agrawal B, Augustin HJ, Dietze GJ. Differential effect of chronic treatment with two beta-blocking agents on insulin sensitivity: the carvedilol-metoprolol study [published erratum appears in J Hypertens 1996;14:1382]. J Hypertens 1996;14:489-94.

71. Giugliano D, Acampora R, Marfella R, De Rosa N, Ziccardi P, Ragone R, et al. Metabolic and cardiovascular effects of carvedilol and atenolol in non-insulin-dependent diabetes mellitus and hypertension: a randomized, controlled trial. Ann Intern Med 1997;126:955-9.

72. Garvey WT, Hermayer KL. Clinical implications of the insulin resistance syndrome. Clin Cornerstone 1998;1:13-28.

73. Pontiroli AE, Pacchioni M, Camisasca R, Lattanzio R. Markers of insulin resistance are associated with cardiovascular morbidity and predict overall mortality in long-standing non-insulin-dependent diabetes mellitus. Acta Diabetol 1998;35:52-6.

74. Lempiainen P, Mykkanen L, Pyorala K, Laakso M, Kuusisto J. Insulin resistance syndrome predicts coronary heart disease events in elderly nondiabetic men. Circulation 1999;100:123-8.

75. Andersson PE, Lithell H. Metabolic effects of doxazosin and enalapril in hypertriglyceridemic, hypertensive men: relationship to changes in skeletal muscle blood flow. Am J Hypertens 1996;9:323-33.

76. Paolisso G, De Riu S, Marrazzo G, Verza M, Varricchio M, D'Onofrio F. Insulin resistance and hyperinsulinemia in patients with chronic congestive heart failure. Metabolism 1991;40:972-7.

77. Swan JW, Walton C, Godsland IF, Clark AL, Coats AJ, Oliver MF. Insulin resistance in chronic heart failure. Eur Heart J 1994;15:1528-32.

78. Swan JW, Anker SD, Walton C, Godsland IF, Clark AL, Leyva F, et al. Insulin resistance in chronic heart failure: relation to severity and etiology of heart failure. J Am Coll Cardiol 1997;30:527-32.

79. Anker SD, Ponikowski PP, Clark AL, Leyva F, Rauchhaus M, Kemp M, et al. Cytokines and neurohormones relating to body composition alterations in the wasting syndrome of chronic heart failure. Eur Heart J 1999;20:683-93.

80. Francis GS, Goldsmith SR, Levine TB, Olivari MT, Cohn JN. The neurohumoral axis in congestive heart failure. Ann Intern Med 1984;101:370-7.

81. Sackner-Bernstein JD. Use of carvedilol in chronic heart failure: challenges in therapeutic management. Prog Cardiovasc Dis 1998;41 Suppl 1:53-8.

82. Packer M, Poole-Wilson PA, Armstrong PW, Cleland JG, Horowitz JD, Massie BM, et al., the ATLAS Study Group. Comparative effects of low and high doses of the angiotensin-converting enzyme inhibitor, lisinopril, on morbidity and mortality in chronic heart failure. Circulation 1999;100:2312-8.

83. Bristow MR, Gilbert EM, Abraham WT, Adams KF, Fowler MB, Hershberger RE, et al., for the MOCHA Investigators. Carvedilol produces dose-related improvements in left ventricular function and survival in subjects with chronic heart failure. Circulation 1996;94:2807-16.

84. Sackner-Bernstein J, Krum H, Goldsmith RL, Kukin ML, Medina N, Yushak M, et al. Should worsening heart failure early after initiation of beta-blocker therapy for chronic heart failure preclude long-term treatment? [Abstract.] Circulation 1995;92:I-395.

85. Krum H, Roecker EB, Mohacsi P, Rouleau JL, Tendera M, Coats AJ, et al., Carvedilol Prospective Randomized Cumulative Survival (COPERNICUS) Study Group. Effects of initiating carvedilol in patients with severe chronic heart failure: results from the COPERNICUS Study. JAMA 2003;289:712-8.

86. Gruppo Italiano per lo Studio della Sopravvivenza nell'infarto Miocardico. GISSI-3: effects of lisinopril and transdermal glyceryl trinitrate singly and together on 6-week mortality and ventricular function after acute myocardial infarction. Lancet 1994;343:1115-22.

87. Køber L, Torp-Pedersen C, Carlsen JE, Bagger H, Eliasen P, Lyngborg K, et al., for the Trandolapril Cardiac Evaluation (TRACE) Study Group. A clinical trial of the angiotensin-converting-enzyme inhibitor trandolapril in patients with left ventricular dysfunction after myocardial infarction. N Engl J Med 1995;333:1670-6.

88. ISIS-4 (Fourth International Study of Infarct Survival) Collaborative Group. ISIS-4: a randomised factorial trial assessing early oral captopril, oral mononitrate, and intravenous magnesium sulphate in 58,050 patients with suspected acute myocardial infarction. Lancet 1995;345:669-85.

89. Anderson TJ, Elstein E, Haber H, Charbonneau F. Comparative study of ACE-inhibition, angiotensin II antagonism, and calcium channel blockade on flow-mediated vasodilation in patients with coronary disease (BANFF study). J Am Coll Cardiol 200;35:60-6.

90. Scholkens BA, Landgraf W. ACE inhibition and atherogenesis. Can J Physiol Pharmacol 2002;80:354-9.

91. Schieffer B, Schieffer E, Hilfiker-Kleiner D, Hilfiker A, Kovanen PT, Kaartinen M, et al. Expression of antiogensin II and interleukin 6 in human coronary atherosclerotic plaques: potential implications for inflammation and plaque instability. Circulation 2000;101:1372-8.

92. Jackson EK, Garrison JC. Renin and angiotensin. In: Hardman JG, Limbird LE, Molinoff PB, Ruddon RW, editors. Goodman and Gilman's the pharmacological basis of therapeutics. 9th ed. New York: McGraw-Hill; 1996. p. 733-58.

93. The NETWORK Investigators. Clinical outcome with enalapril in symptomatic chronic heart failure; a dose comparison. Eur Heart J 1998;19:481-9.

94. Fogari R, Zoppi A, Corradi L, Lazzari P, Mugellini A, Lusardi P. Comparative effects of lisinopril and losartan on insulin sensitivity in the treatment of non diabetic hypertensive patients. Br J Clin Pharmacol 1998;46:467-71.

95. Pollare T, Lithell H, Berne C. A comparison of the effects of hydrochlorothiazide and captopril on glucose and lipid metabolism in patients with hypertension. N Engl J Med 1989;321:868-73.

96. Hunter SJ, Wiggam MI, Ennis CN, Whitehead HM, Sheridan B, Atkinson AB, et al. Comparison of effects of captopril used either alone or in combination with a thiazide diuretic on insulin action in hypertensive Type 2 diabetic patients: a double-blind crossover study. Diabet Med 1999;16:482-7.

97. Weinberger MH. Mechanisms of diuretic effects on carbohydrate tolerance, insulin sensitivity and lipid levels. Eur Heart J 1992;13 Suppl G:5-9.

98. Tomiyama H, Kushiro T, Abeta H, Ishii T, Takahashi A, Furukawa L, et al. Kinins contribute to the improvement of insulin sensitivity during treatment with angiotensin converting enzyme inhibitor. Hypertension 1994;23:450-5.

99. Janssen JJ, Gans RO, van der Meulen J, Pijpers R, ter Wee PM. Comparison between the effects of amlodipine and lisinopril on proteinuria in nondiabetic renal failure: a double-blind, randomized prospective study. Am J Hypertens 1998;11:1074-9.

100. Brenner BM, Cooper ME, de Zeeuw D, Keane WF, Mitch WE, Parving HH, et al., for the RENAAL Study Investigators. Effects of losartan on renal and cardiovascular outcomes in patients with type 2 diabetes and nephropathy. N Engl J Med 2001;345:861-9.

101. Lewis EJ, Hunsicker LG, Clarke WR, Berl T, Pohl MA, Lewis JB, et al., for the Collaborative Study Group. Renoprotective effect of the angiotensin-receptor antagonist irbesartan in patients with nephropathy due to type 2 diabetes. N Engl J Med 2001;345:851-60.

102. Packer M, Lee WH, Medina N, Yushak M, Kessler PD. Functional renal insufficiency during long-term therapy with captopril and enalapril in severe chronic heart failure. Ann Intern Med 1987;106:346-54.

103. Massie BM, Kramer BL, Topic N. Lack of relationship between the short-term hemodynamic effects of captopril and subsequent clinical responses. Circulation 1984;69:1135-41.

104. Captopril Multicenter Research Group. A placebo-controlled trial of captopril in refractory chronic congestive heart failure. J Am Coll Cardiol 1983;2:755-63.

105. Lee WH, Packer M. Prognostic importance of serum sodium concentration and its modification by converting-enzyme inhibition in patients with severe chronic heart failure. Circulation 1986;73:257-67.

106. Packer M, Lee WH, Medina N, Yushak M, Kessler PD, Gottlieb SS. Influence of diabetes mellitus on changes in left ventricular performance and renal function produced by converting enzyme inhibition in patients with severe chronic heart failure. Am J Med 1987;82:1119-26.

107. Dzau VJ, Hollenberg NK. Renal response to captopril in severe heart failure: role of furosemide in natriuresis and reversal of hyponatremia. Ann Intern Med 1984;100:777-82.

108. Packer M, Lee WH, Medina N, Yushak M, Kessler P. Identification of patients with severe heart failure most likely to fail long-term therapy with converting-enzyme inhibitors [abstract]. J Am Coll Cardiol 1986;7:181A.

109. Burnier M, Brunner HR. Angiotensin II receptor antagonists. Lancet 2000;355:637-45.

110. Baruch L, Anand I, Cohen IS, Ziesche S, Judd D, Cohn JN, for the Vasodilator Heart Failure Trial (V-HeFT) Study Group. Augmented short- and long-term hemodynamic and hormonal effects of an angiotensin receptor blocker added to angiotensin converting enzyme inhibitor therapy in patients with heart failure. Circulation 1999;99:2658-64.

111. Havranek EP, Thomas I, Smith WB, Ponce GA, Bilsker M, Munger MA, et al. Dose-related beneficial long-term hemodynamic and clinical efficacy of irbesartan in heart failure. J Am Coll Cardiol 1999;33:1174-81.

112. MacFadyen RJ, Lee AF, Morton JJ, Pringle SD, Struthers AD. How often are angiotensin II and aldosterone concentrations raised during chronic ACE inhibitor treatment in cardiac failure? Heart 1999;82:57-61.

113. Roig E, Perez-Villa F, Morales M, Jiménez W, Orús J, Heras M, et al. Clinical implications of increased plasma angiotensin II despite ACE inhibitor therapy in patients with congestive heart failure. Eur Heart J 2000;21:53-7.

114. Pitt B, Segal R, Martinez FA, Meurers G, Cowley AJ, Thomas I, et al., the ELITE Study Investigators. Randomised trial of losartan versus captopril in patients over 65 with heart failure (Evaluation of Losartan in the Elderly Study, ELITE). Lancet 1997;349:747-52.

115. Pitt B, Poole-Wilson PA, Segal R, Martinez FA, Dickstein K, Camm AJ, et al. Effect of losartan compared with captopril on mortality in patients with symptomatic heart failure: randomised trial—the Losartan Heart Failure Survival Study ELITE II. Lancet 2000;355:1582-7.

116. McKelvie RS, Yusuf S, Pericak D, Avezum A, Burns RJ, Probstfield J, et al. Comparison of candesartan, enalapril, and their combination in congestive heart failure: randomized evaluation of strategies for left ventricular dysfunction (RESOLVD) pilot study. The RESOLVD Pilot Study Investigators. Circulation 1999;100:1056-64.

117. Weber KT, Villarreal D. Aldosterone and antialdosterone therapy in congestive heart failure. Am J Cardiol 1993;71:3A-11A.

118. Lindenfeld J, Robertson AD, Lowes BD, Bristow MR, MOCHA Investigators. Aspirin impairs reverse myocardial remodeling in patients with heart failure treated with beta-blockers. J Am Coll Cardiol 2001;38:1950-6.

119. Tuzcu EM, Kapadia SR, Tutar E, Ziada KM, Hobbs RE, McCarthy PM, et al. High prevalence of coronary atherosclerosis in asymptomatic teenagers and young adults: evidence from intravascular ultrasound. Circulation 2001;103:2705-10.

120. Gattis WA, O'Connor CM, Gheorghiade M. The Initiation Management Predischarge Process for Assessment of Carvedilol Therapy for Heart Failure (IMPACT-HF) Study: design and implications. Rev Cardiovasc Med 2002;3 Suppl 3:S48-54.

121. Chobanian AV, Bakris GL, Black HR, Cushman WC, Green LA, Izzo JL Jr, et al. The Seventh Report of the Joint National Committee on Prevention, Detection, Evaluation, and Treatment of High Blood Pressure: the JNC 7 report [published erratum appears in JAMA 2003;290:197]. JAMA 2003;289:2560-72.

122. Lewington S, Clarke R, Qizilbash N, Peto R, Collins R, Prospective Studies Collaboration. Age-specific relevance of usual blood pressure to vascular mortality: a meta-analysis of individual data for one million adults in 61 prospective studies [published erratum appears in Lancet 2003;361:1060]. Lancet 2002;360:1903-13.

123. Svensson P, de Faire U, Sleight P, Yusuf S, Ostergren J. Comparative effects of ramipril on ambulatory and office blood pressures: a HOPE Substudy. Hypertension 2001;38:E28-32.

124. National Cholesterol Education Program. Third Report of the Expert Panel on Detection, Evaluation, and Treatment of High Blood Cholesterol in Adults (Adult Treatment Panel III): final report. September 2002. Retrieved August 29, 2003, from the World Wide Web: http://www.nhlbi.nih.gov/guidelines/cholesterol/atp3_rpt.htm.

125. Heart Protection Study Collaborative Group. MRC/BHF Heart Protection Study of cholesterol-lowering with simvastatin in 5963 people with diabetes: a randomised placebo-controlled trial. Lancet 2003;361:2005-16.

126. Cleland JG. Is aspirin "the weakest link" in cardiovascular prophylaxis? The surprising lack of evidence supporting the use of aspirin for cardiovascular disease. Prog Cardiovasc Dis 2002;44:275-92.

127. Adler AI, Stratton IM, Neil HA, Yudkin JS, Matthews DR, Cull CA, et al. Association of systolic blood pressure with macrovascular and microvascular complications of type 2 diabetes (UKPDS 36): prospective observational study. BMJ 2000;321:412-9.

128. Centers for Disease Control and Prevention. National diabetes fact sheet: general information and national estimates on diabetes in the United States, 2000. Atlanta (GA): U.S. Department of Health and Human Services, Centers for Disease Control and Prevention, 2002. Retrieved August 29, 2003, from the World Wide Web: http://www.diabetes.org/main/info/facts/facts_natl.jsp.

129. Diabetes Prevention Program Research Group. Reduction in the incidence of type 2 diabetes with lifestyle intervention or metformin. N Engl J Med 2002;346:393-403.

130. Heart Protection Study Collaborative Group. MRC/BHF Heart Protection Study of cholesterol lowering with simvastatin in 20,536 high-risk individuals: a randomised placebo-controlled trial. Lancet 2002;360:7-22.

CHAPTER 2

Cardiac Resynchronization Therapy

David L. Hayes, MD

Early Pacing Studies

In the early 1990s, right-sided atrioventricular (AV) sequential (dual-chamber) pacing with short AV delay was proposed as empirical therapy to relieve the symptoms of congestive heart failure in patients with severe left ventricular dysfunction.[1] Hochleitner et al.[1] published one of the earliest reports of pacing for the treatment of idiopathic dilated cardiomyopathy with short AV interval DDD pacing. In this uncontrolled study, Hochleitner et al. treated 16 patients critically ill with idiopathic dilated cardiomyopathy refractory to pharmacologic therapy who were in New York Heart Association (NYHA) functional class III or IV. The authors reported dramatic improvement in NYHA functional class and a reduction in mortality from that expected at 1 year. The same group subsequently published the 5-year follow-up results for their original patient cohort.[2] No deaths occurred because of continued deterioration in ventricular function, and no patient needed rehospitalization because of worsening heart failure after pacemaker implantation.

Subsequent investigators demonstrated markedly discrepant responses to standard dual-chamber pacing, with great interindividual variability and no consistent benefit from dual-chamber pacing.[3-6] The hemodynamic improvement was found to be related to optimal synchronization of atrial and ventricular contractions[7] (Fig. 1).

However, predominantly patients with prolonged PR intervals appeared to benefit from dual-chamber pacing, that is, those whose atrial contraction occurs so prematurely that the atrial "kick" to ventricular contraction is lost. Subsequently, clinical trials showed that dual-chamber pacing had limited long-term efficacy.[4-6]

Largely on the basis of these data, and despite their limitations, pacing for the treatment of medically refractory dilated cardiomyopathy was designated a class IIb indication for pacing in the 1998 American College of Cardiology and American Heart Association (ACC/AHA) guidelines.[8]

39

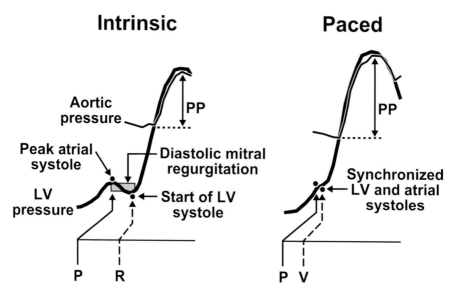

Figure 1. Left ventricular (LV) hemodynamic tracing without optimized atrioventricular (AV) synchrony (Intrinsic) (left) and after AV interval optimization (Paced) (right). With optimization, left atrial and LV systoles are synchronized, maximum effective preload is achieved, and diastolic mitral regurgitation is minimized. PP, pulse pressure; R, intrinsic ventricular depolarization; V, paced ventricular event. (From Auricchio A, et al. Association between preload and optimal pacing mode in CHF patients. Heart Failure Society of America 1998. By permission of Guidant Corporation.)

Mechanical and Hemodynamic Consequences of Left Bundle Branch Block

When optimization of AV synchrony failed to produce clinical improvement in a substantial portion of patients with congestive heart failure, the need for correction of intraventricular conduction disturbances and whether this might result in clinical improvement were considered. Although estimates from limited studies vary on the proportion of patients with heart failure who also have ventricular dyssynchrony—usually left bundle branch—the number is large (27% to 53%) and certainly in excess of the rate in the general population.[9-12]

The duration of QRS has been shown to correlate with mortality, that is, the greater the duration, the higher the mortality[13,14] (Fig. 2). In addition to the higher mortality these conduction abnormalities cause, mechanical dyssynchrony between the left ventricle and right ventricle throughout the cardiac cycle can adversely affect left ventricular performance.[15,16] To understand the principles of cardiac resynchronization therapy (CRT), the mechanical and hemodynamic effects of left bundle branch block (LBBB) need to be reviewed.

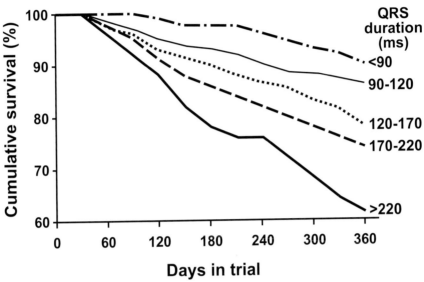

Figure 2. From the VEST study, analysis of 3,654 electrocardiograms from patients in New York Heart Association class II-IV. The relative risk of mortality in the group with the widest QRS was 5 times greater than that of the group with the narrowest QRS. According to this study, age, creatinine level, left ventricular ejection fraction, heart rate, and QRS duration were independent predictors of mortality. (From Gottipaty et al.[13] By permission of the American College of Cardiology.)

Ventricular Activation

Normal electrical activation of the ventricles is conducted by the His bundle and Purkinje system. The activation spreads transmurally from the endocardium to multiple paraseptal epicardial regions, resulting in synchronous contraction of the ventricles. The latest epicardial activation occurs over the anterior or inferior base of the right side of the heart.[17] In LBBB, the left ventricle is activated belatedly through the septum from the right ventricle, with anteroseptal crossing preceding inferoseptal crossing, and the latest activation is in the inferior aspect of the left ventricle, often remote from the base.[18]

Interventricular Dyssynchrony

In patients with LBBB, the delay between the onset of contraction of the left ventricle and right ventricle is significant, but without LBBB, there is no significant difference.[15] LBBB is associated with significantly later opening and closing of the aortic valve and later opening of the mitral valve, but it does not affect the timing of right ventricular events (Fig. 3). This leads to a reversal of the usual sequence of

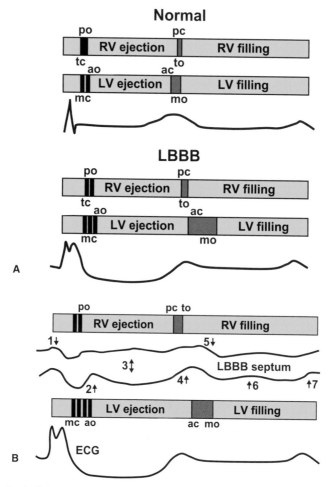

Figure 3. A, Relation between right ventricular (RV) and left ventricular (LV) events in, top, normal subjects and, bottom, patients with left bundle branch block (LBBB). In the normal group, LV events either precede or occur simultaneously with the RV events. In LBBB, the sequence is reversed. Times of pulmonic (po), tricuspid (to), aortic (ao), and mitral valve opening (mo) and closings (pc, tc, ac, and mc, respectively) are indicated. B, Effect of LBBB on interventricular septal motion and the relation to dynamic interventricular asynchrony. 1, RV contraction in LBBB patients occurring earlier than LV systole and being associated with an abrupt displacement of the interventricular septum into the LV; 2, pulmonic ejection occurring during ventricular isovolumic systole and associated with septal displacement toward the RV; 3, septal motion usually flat or paradoxic during simultaneous RV and LV contraction; 4, continuation of LV systole after pc and association with displacement of the septum into the RV; 5, with tricuspid valve opening (to), the septum is displaced toward the LV; 6, septal displacement reversed with mo; 7, during atrial systole, the septum is further displaced. (From Grines et al.[15] By permission of the American Heart Association.)

right ventricular and left ventricular systole and diastole, with dynamic interventricular dyssynchrony throughout the cardiac cycle. The delay in aortic valve closure leads to a relative decrease in the duration of left ventricular filling. In patients with LBBB, delayed depolarization or abnormal repolarization may result in regional myocardial contraction extending into early diastole, causing a delay of mitral valve opening and shortened left ventricular filling time.[15]

Most patients with LBBB have abnormal motion of the ventricular septum, which is probably related to the interventricular dyssynchrony and the resulting abnormal pressure gradient between left and right ventricles.[15] Because of the abnormal septal motion, left ventricular end-systolic diameter is increased significantly and regional septal ejection fraction is decreased significantly with LBBB. LBBB in patients with or without cardiac disease can decrease global left ventricular ejection fraction (LVEF), cardiac output, mean arterial pressure, and the ratio of change in pressure to change in time (dP/dt).[15,19]

In summary, the heterogeneous activation and altered repolarization lead to a decreased preload and a reduced mechanically effective muscle mass. The abnormal physiologic effects that result from LBBB are indicated in Figure 4.

It should be noted that the electrocardiographic findings consistent with LBBB may not represent a true electrical blockage of the entire left bundle but some

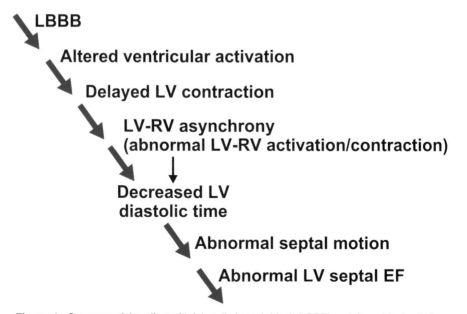

Figure 4. Summary of the effect of left bundle branch block (LBBB) on left ventricular (LV) function. EF, ejection fraction; RV, right ventricular.

variation of the intramyocardial conduction abnormality. This could explain some of the heterogeneity seen clinically in response to resynchronization.

Application of Cardiac Resynchronization Therapy

Mechanisms

The mechanisms by which cardiac resynchronization can improve left ventricular function and produce functional improvement in patients with congestive heart failure are complex. The following mechanisms should be considered:

- Acute hemodynamic changes that result in improved left ventricular efficiency
- Improvement of intraventricular dyssynchrony
- Improvement of interventricular dyssynchrony
- Improvement of "intrawall" dyssynchrony
- Reverse remodeling of the left ventricle
- Reverse remodeling of the left atrium
- Reduction in mitral regurgitation
- Normalization of neurohumoral factors
- Improved cardiovascular autonomic control (normalization of the standard deviation of averaged normal-to-normal heartbeats [SDANN])

Cardiac resynchronization can reduce the mechanical *interventricular* dyssynchrony between the right and left ventricles that may be induced by any interventricular conduction delay. As noted above, LBBB is the most common interventricular conduction delay in most cardiomyopathic states. Most of the data available have been collected from patients with LBBB. Although few data are available about patients with right bundle branch block (RBBB) and class III or IV heart failure, their response to cardiac resynchronization does not appear to differ from that of patients with LBBB.[20]

The reduction of *intraventricular* dyssynchrony within the left ventricle associated with LBBB appears more important. Minimizing intraventricular dyssynchrony has been shown to improve global left ventricular function and result in functional improvement. Pacing only from specific left ventricular sites may also reduce abnormal left ventricular activation and improve left ventricular contraction efficiency.[21-23] In an acute pacing study, Kass et al.[21] used intraventricular manometry to compare pacing from the right ventricular apex, right ventricular septum pacing, biventricular pacing, and left ventricular pacing only. As shown in Figure 5, there was no significant difference in pressure volume loops when pacing from the right ventricular sites. Left ventricular contraction improved with pacing in biventricular and left ventricular configurations. In this relatively small group of patients, left ventricular pacing only resulted in better hemodynamic improvement than biventricular pacing.

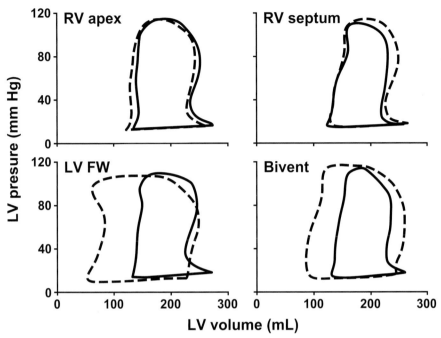

Figure 5. Pressure volume loops from an acute pacing study with pacing from different sites (dashed line) vs. normal sinus rhythm (solid line). Upper left, Pacing from right ventricular (RV) apex; upper right, pacing from RV septum; lower left, left ventricular (LV) pacing; lower right, biventricular (Bivent) pacing. Greatest improvement was with LV pacing configurations, and LV only was better than the biventricular configuration. FW, free wall. (From Kass et al.[21] By permission of the American Heart Association.)

Earlier work for the Pacing Therapies for Congestive Heart Failure (PATH-CHF) I study demonstrated that improvement in left ventricular efficiency, dP/dt, and pulse pressure was greatest when the left ventricle was paced from the mid-lateral wall (Fig. 6). Although this general principle may apply in many patients, other left ventricular pacing sites may be optimal for patients with left ventricular regional wall motion abnormalities.

Not only may interventricular dyssynchrony be responsible for many of the symptoms of patients with congestive heart failure but more recent data also implicate "intrawall" dyssynchrony (i.e., dyssynchronous contraction within the septal or lateral wall) as a contributing factor.[24] The degree to which the surface QRS reflects the status of interventricular dyssynchrony is unclear. To date, CRT trials have included a wide QRS as an inclusion criterion. Most clinicians have observed the dyssynchronous contraction that occurs on an echocardiogram or multigated acquisition nuclear scan in a patient with LBBB. Intuitively, it is understandable that

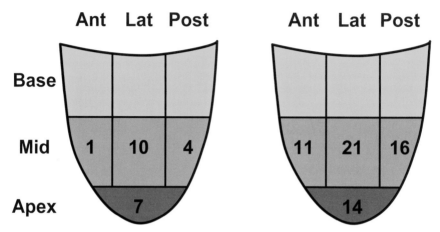

Figure 6. Left, The left ventricular diagram shows the percentage change in pulse pressure when pacing from various regions of the left ventricle. The greatest improvement occurred when pacing from the mid-lateral wall. Right, The percentage change in left ventricular dP/dt when pacing from various regions of the left ventricle. The greatest improvement occurred when pacing from the mid-lateral wall. Ant, anterior; Lat, lateral; Post, posterior. (From Auricchio et al.[22] By permission of Excerpta Medica.)

notable dyssynchrony accompanies LBBB. It is more difficult to understand how clinically important dyssynchrony occurs in a patient with a normal surface QRS. Patients with clinical congestive heart failure and a normal surface QRS complex have been shown by tissue Doppler imaging (TDI) to have clinically important interventricular dyssynchrony.[25,26] This leads to the question of whether QRS width should be used as a selection criterion or whether another technique, most likely TDI would better identify which patients have clinically important interventricular dyssynchrony as an indication for cardiac resynchronization. CRT trials have demonstrated changes in echocardiographic parameters consistent with left ventricular reverse remodeling, including a reduction in left ventricular end-systolic and end-diastolic dimensions. Although it is assumed that the reverse remodeling is due at least partly to chronic changes resulting from resynchronization, acute changes in left ventricular function have also been demonstrated. Several investigators have demonstrated acute changes in left ventricular efficiency as evidenced by an increase in left ventricular dP/dt. It appears that both acute hemodynamic and chronic "remodeling" are responsible for the improvement seen with resynchronization.

There also is evidence that sudden death in patients with heart failure is correlated with left ventricular size[27] (Fig. 7). Multiple studies have shown that CRT results in a decrease in left ventricular end-diastolic dimensions[28,29] (Fig. 8). A

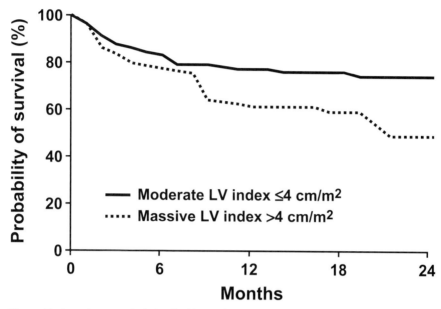

Figure 7. Long-term survival stratified by moderate and massive left ventricular (LV) index. Patients with a massive LV index had significantly higher mortality. (Modified from Lee et al.[27] By permission of Excerpta Medica.)

decrease in left ventricular mass has also been demonstrated by echocardiographic techniques[28] (Fig. 9).

A reduction in functional mitral regurgitation is often seen after resynchronization is applied.[30-33] Initially reported in nonrandomized observational studies,[30,31] the reduction of functional mitral regurgitation has also been demonstrated in controlled trials.[32,33] It is important to distinguish between functional mitral regurgitation and structural mitral valve disease. There is no evidence that resynchronization will favorably alter mitral regurgitation in a patient with structural disease. Some physicians consider structural mitral valve disease with any notable degree of regurgitation as a relative contraindication to CRT and instead consider it a target for surgical correction. However, in many cases, it may be difficult to distinguish between functional mitral regurgitation and structural mitral regurgitation, particularly in the presence of coexistent annular dilatation.

As with general functional improvement and improvement in left ventricular efficiency, reduction in functional mitral regurgitation is related to acute hemodynamic and longer term reverse remodeling (Fig. 10). As left ventricular contraction is resynchronized, the rate of rise of left ventricular systolic pressure, left ventricular dP/dt increases, which in turn leads to an increase in transmitral pressure gradient and

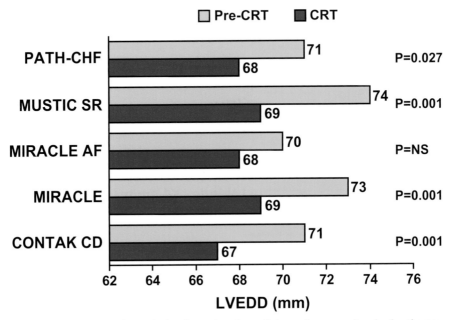

Figure 8. Change in left ventricular dimensions in multiple cardiac resynchronization therapy (CRT) studies. All the studies consistently demonstrated left ventricular reverse remodeling. LVEDD, left ventricular end-diastolic dimension. NS, not significant.

a decrease in functional mitral regurgitation.[33] Longer term, as left ventricular end-systolic and end-diastolic volumes decrease, there is a corresponding decrease in end-systolic and end-diastolic dimensions (Fig. 11). Also, less stretch of the mitral valve annulus as a result of the decrease in ventricular dimensions is thought to contribute mechanically to the decrease in mitral regurgitation.

A secondary effect of the decrease in mitral regurgitation and left ventricular dimensions is the decrease in left atrial dimension. According to anecdotal reports and limited information (i.e., abstract form), some patients with chronic atrial fibrillation that responds to cardiac resynchronization can revert to normal sinus rhythm. The current belief is that a return to normal sinus rhythm from chronic atrial fibrillation should not be expected. Theoretically, cardiac resynchronization could prevent paroxysmal atrial fibrillation in a patient with congestive heart failure from progressing to chronic atrial fibrillation; data are beginning to emerge but are not yet available.

There are limited data to suggest that cardiac resynchronization may lead to a decrease in ventricular arrhythmias.[34] Cardiac resynchronization may decrease wall stress and ventricular size; change conduction patterns; affect metalloproteinases and the extracellular matrix, gap junction protein function, and ion channel

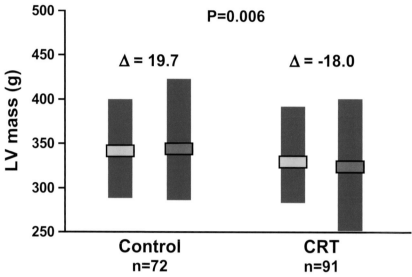

Figure 9. Data from the MIRACLE trial demonstrating a reduction in left ventricular (LV) mass measured echocardiographically support the concept of reverse remodeling. CRT, cardiac resynchronization therapy. Yellow rectangles, baseline; red rectangles, 6 months. (Courtesy of Medtronic.)

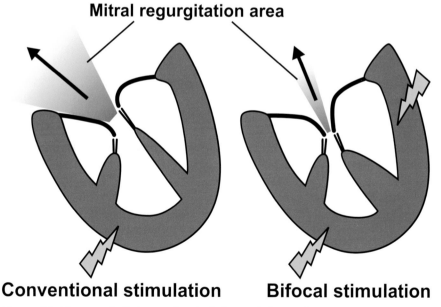

Figure 10. Diagram of mitral regurgitant jet before and after cardiac resynchronization. (Courtesy of Jose C. Pachon, MD.)

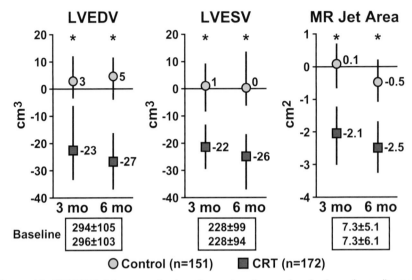

Figure 11. MIRACLE data comparing baseline and post-resynchronization echocardiographic results. The decrease in left ventricular end-diastolic volume (LVEDV) and left ventricular end-systolic volume (LVESV) correlates with a significant decrease in the mitral regurgitant (MR) jet. *, $P<0.001$. CRT, cardiac resynchronization therapy. (From St. John Sutton et al.[32] By permission of the American Heart Association.)

function; and decrease the sympathetic and neurohormonal factors that may promote ventricular arrhythmias.

The data are convincing for a correlation between survival and norepinephrine levels in patients with congestive heart failure[35] (Fig. 12). Although preliminary results suggested a normalization of norepinephrine levels, this was not borne out at the completion of the study.[36] More recently, resynchronization studies have shown a reduction in brain natriuretic peptide.[37]

CRT may restore autonomic balance in heart failure as evidenced by restoration of heart rate variability or SDANN.[38] A loss of SDANN has been shown to correlate with higher mortality.[39] Whether cardiac resynchronization will consistently improve heart rate variability and, more importantly, whether it is clinically important in this group of patients are not known.

Clinical Results

Patients With Normal Sinus Rhythm

Clinical work with CRT dates to 1993. Several acute and uncontrolled or observational chronic studies and the clinical variables that improved are summarized in Table 1.

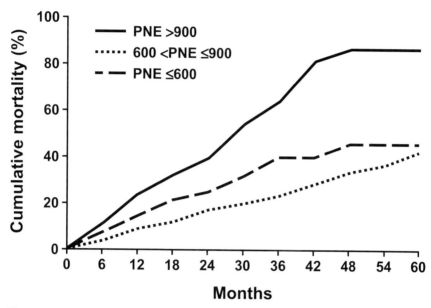

Figure 12. Survival curves for heart failure patients with specified plasma levels of norepinephrine (PNE). Patients with the highest levels, PNE >900, had the worst survival. (From Francis et al.[35] By permission of the American Heart Association.)

Numerous randomized clinical trials have been completed (Table 2), and some trials are still ongoing.

The PATH-CHF I study is a single-blind, randomized, crossover, controlled trial designed to evaluate acute hemodynamic function and to assess long-term clinical benefit of right ventricular, left ventricular, and biventricular pacing in patients with moderate to severe congestive heart failure and interventricular conduction block.[48] Twenty-seven patients were studied. Aortic pulse pressure and dP/dt were measured at baseline and during acute pacing. Biventricular and left ventricular pacing increased dP/dt and pulse pressure more than right ventricular pacing ($P<0.01$), and left ventricular pacing increased dP/dt more than biventricular pacing ($P<0.01$). Also, pulse pressure and dP/dt increased at a patient-specific optimal AV delay in 20 patients with a wide QRS duration (180±22 milliseconds). Short AV delays decreased dP/dt and pulse pressure in five patients with a narrower QRS duration (128±12 milliseconds).

In a substudy, the hemodynamic effects of varying the ventricle-to-ventricle (VV) interval were assessed. An offset of 20 to 80 milliseconds between left and right ventricular stimulation produced a greater change in dP/dt than simultaneous biventricular stimulation. Other investigators have also demonstrated the significance of VV offset in certain patients[49] (Fig. 13).

Table 1. Observational Trials of Cardiac Resynchronization Therapy in Congestive Heart Failure

Author	Patients	Improvement
Cazeau et al.[40]	Six-week technical feasibility study of 4-chamber pacing in a 54-year-old with NYHA class IV heart failure, LBBB, 200-ms PR interval, and interatrial conduction delay	Yes—clinical status
Foster et al.[41]	Acute study of biventricular pacing in 18 postoperative coronary revascularization patients	Yes—hemodynamics
Cazeau et al.[42]	Eight patients with wide QRS and end-stage heart failure, compared effect of various ventricular pacing sites (RV apex, RVOT, RV apex-LV pacing, RVOT-LV pacing), follow-up, 3-17 mo	Yes—hemodynamics & functional status, in patients with LV or biventricular pacing only
Blanc et al.[43]	Acute hemodynamic study comparing effect of various ventricular pacing sites (RV apex, RVOT, LV, or biventricular pacing) in 27 patients with severe heart failure with 1° AV block and/or IVCD	Yes—hemodynamics in patients with LV or biventricular pacing only
Kass et al.[21]	Acute hemodynamic study comparing effect of various ventricular pacing modes (RV apex, RV septal, LV free wall, or biventricular pacing) in 18 patients with advanced heart failure	Yes—hemodynamics in patients with LV or biventricular pacing only
Saxon et al.[23]	Study of biventricular pacing in 11 postoperative cardiac surgery patients with depressed LV function	Yes—hemodynamics
Gras et al.[44]	European and Canadian multicenter trial of biventricular pacing in 68 patients with dilated cardiomyopathy, IVCD, and NYHA class III/IV heart failure (InSync Study, interim results, 3-mo follow-up)	Yes—QOL, NYHA class, 6-min hall walk distance

Table 1 (continued)

Author	Patients	Improvement
Leclercq et al.[45]	Acute hemodynamic study comparing single-site RV DDD pacing with biventricular pacing in 18 patients with NYHA class III/IV heart failure	Yes—hemodynamics for biventricular pacing only
Gras et al.[46]	Included 117 patients (103 successfully implanted with CRT device) with idiopathic or ischemic dilated cardiomyopathy, NYHA class III/IV heart failure, LV dysfunction, and IVCD (InSync Study, final analysis, long-term follow-up)	Yes—QOL, NYHA class, 6-min hall walk distance

AV, atrioventricular; CRT, cardiac resynchronization therapy; IVCD, intraventricular conduction defect; LBBB, left bundle branch block; LV, left ventricular; NYHA, New York Heart Association; QOL, quality-of-life score; RV, right ventricular; RVOT, right ventricular outflow tract.
From Abraham WT, Hayes DL. Cardiac resynchronization for heart failure. Circulation 2003;108:2596-603. By permission of the American Heart Association.

Assessment at 12 months' follow-up showed a statistically significant improvement in several variables (Table 3).

In a study in which patients received CRT for 4 weeks "on," 4 weeks "off," then back to 4 weeks "on," the assessed end points deteriorated when CRT was turned "off." An example of the peak $\dot{V}O_2$ data from this study is shown in Figure 14, which also shows the study design.

Reverse remodeling of the left ventricle was demonstrated by a statistically significant decrease in end-systolic and end-diastolic volumes.

Multisite Stimulation in Cardiomyopathy (MUSTIC) was a randomized crossover (3 months) single-blinded, biventricular VDD vs. "no pacing" trial, with the primary end point of a 6-minute walk and secondary end points of quality of life, peak $\dot{V}O_2$, hospital admissions, congestive heart failure, total mortality, and patient preference for pacing mode.[50] After patients were selected for the study, they were followed for 1 month before randomization. Each phase of the study was for 3 months. Patients were randomly assigned to CRT vs. no CRT. Inclusion criteria included normal sinus rhythm-no indication for pacing, NYHA class III congestive heart failure, optimized drug therapy, LVEF less than 35%, left ventricular end-diastolic dimension more than 60 mm, intraventricular conduction defect (QRS width

Table 2. Controlled Clinical Trials in Pacing for Congestive Heart Failure (CHF)

Study	Patient inclusion criteria	End point(s)	Treatment arms	Key results
MIRACLE	NYHA class III/IV on stable drug regimen LVEDD ≥55 mm, LVEF ≤35% QRS width ≥130 ms	QOL NYHA class Six-min hall walk	Randomized to pacing or no pacing for 6 mo	Sustained improvement in all 3 end points
PATH-CHF NYHA class II-IV	DCM of any cause on stable drug regimen QRS ≥120 ms	Acute: Maximum LV pressure derivative, aortic pulse pressure Chronic: QOL, NYHA class, 6-min hall walk, hospitalizations	Acute hemodynamic assessment of RV pacing LV pacing vs. BiV pacing Chronic: randomized to CRT vs. no CRT with crossover	Acute: BiV and LV—↑LV pressure derivative & aortic pulse pressure more than RV pacing LV pacing— ↑LV pressure derivative more than BiV pacing Chronic: Improvement in 6-min hall walk, QOL, NYHA final class
MUSTIC-NSR	NYHA class III Refractory symptoms on stable drug therapy LVEF <35% LVEDD >60 mm Six-min hall walk <450 m NSR with QRS >150 ms	QOL, 6-min hall walk, peak $\dot{V}O_2$ Hospital admission for CHF	BiV pacing vs. No pacing with crossover	Sustained improvement in all end points Fewer hospital admissions with CRT

Table 2 (continued)

Study	Patient inclusion criteria	End point(s)	Treatment arms	Key results
MUSTIC-AF	NYHA class III Refractory symptoms on stable drug therapy LVEF <35% LVEDD >60 mm Six-min hall walk <450 m AF with paced QRS >200 ms	QOL, 6-min hall walk, peak $\dot{V}O_2$, hospitalization Hospital admission for CHF	BiV pacing *vs.* No pacing with crossover	Sustained improvement in all end points Fewer hospital admissions with CRT
InSync III	NYHA class III/IV on stable drug regimen LVEDD ≥60 mm, LVEF ≤35% QRS width ≥130 ms	QOL NYHA class Six-min hall walk	BiV pacing with optimized AV and VV intervals *vs.* No pacing with crossover	Sustained improvement in all end points
CARE-HF	NYHA class III/IV on stable drug regimen LVEDD ≥60 mm, LVEF ≤35% QRS width ≥150 ms or >120 ms with echo study	Mortality QOL Economic outcomes Echo variables Neurohormonal measurements	BiV pacing *vs.* No pacing with crossover	Enrollment completed (3/03)
VecToR	NYHA class III/ IV LVEF ≤35% QRS ≥140 ms LVEDD >54 mm	QOL Mortality Echo variables	BiV pacing *vs.* No pacing with crossover	In progress
ReLeVent	NYHA class III/IV LVEF <35% QRS >140 ms LVEDD >55 mm	Six-min hall walk LVEDD LVESD Mortality QOL	BiV pacing *vs.* No pacing with crossover	In progress

Table 2 (continued)

Study	Patient inclusion criteria	End point(s)	Treatment arms	Key results
MUSTIC-II	NYHA class III/IV AF S/P ablation and paced for >3 mo LVEDD >60 mm QRS >200 ms Six-min hall walk <450 m LVEF <35%	Exercise tolerance QOL Hospitalization rates Modification of drug therapy	BiV pacing *vs.* No pacing with cross-over	In progress
MIRACLE ICD[47]	LVEF ≤35% LVEDD >55 mm NYHA class III/IV(cohort in class II also enrolled) IVCD (QRS >130 ms) Indication for ICD	QOL NYHA class Six-min hall walk Efficacy anti-tachycardia therapy with BiV pacing	Pacing *vs.* No pacing for 6 mo	Improved QOL, functional status, exercise capacity Normal ICD function

AF, atrial fibrillation; BiV, biventricular; CRT, cardiac resynchronization therapy; DCM, dilated cardiomyopathy; echo, echocardiographic; ICD, implantable cardioverter-defibrillator; IVCD, intraventricular conduction defect; LV, left ventricular; LVEDD, left ventricular end-diastolic dimension; LVEF, left ventricular ejection fraction; LVESD, left ventricular end-systolic dimension; NSR, normal sinus rhythm; NYHA, New York Heart Association; QOL, quality-of-life score; RV, right ventricular; S/P, status post.

Table 3. PATH-CHF I Comparison of Variables Assessed at Baseline and 12 Months

Variable	Patients, no.	Baseline	12 months	P value
$\dot{V}O_2$ max, mL/kg per min	22	12.6±0.6	15.6±0.9	<0.001
$\dot{V}O_2$ AT	21	9.9±0.5	11.5±0.6	0.037
Six-min hall walk, m	25	357±20	446±15	<0.001
Quality-of-life score	28	49±4	20±4	<0.001
NYHA functional class	29	3.1	1.9	<0.001

AT, anaerobic threshold; NYHA, New York Heart Association.

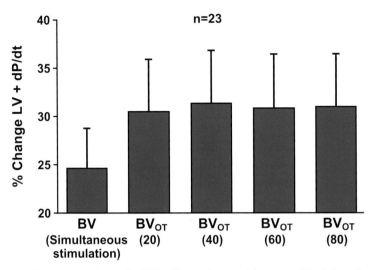

Figure 13. Percentage change in dP/dt with varying ventricle-to-ventricle timing. An offset of 20 to 80 ms resulted in greater hemodynamic improvement than simultaneous biventricular (BV) stimulation. LV, left ventricular; OT, offset time. (Data from Butter C, Auricchio A, Stellbrink C, Ding J, Doelger A, Huvelle E, et al. Biventricular resynchronization therapy for heart failure patients: does longer LV-RV conduction delay always yield better hemodynamic responses? [Abstract.] Pacing Clin Electrophysiol 2001;24:629.)

>150 milliseconds), and a 6-minute hall walk less than 450 meters. Sixty-seven patients in normal sinus rhythm with NYHA functional class III status were enrolled in the study. The improvement shown in all end points at 12 months was maintained at 24 months (Table 4). In this study, 85% of the patients felt better when the biventricular pacemaker was on—an important fact for physicians to know.

The change in left ventricular end-diastolic volume for MUSTIC is shown in Figure 8. Changes in the 6-minute hall walk, quality-of-life score, peak $\dot{V}O_2$, and NYHA functional class are shown in Figures 15 to 18.

The InSync (Multicenter InSync Randomized Clinical Evaluation [MIRACLE]) trial was a double-blind controlled randomized study.[28] Initially, the 532 patients were randomly assigned to biventricular pacing or "no" pacing for 6 months. At 6 months, all patients received biventricular pacing. Inclusion criteria included patients with NYHA functional class III or IV heart failure, LVEF of 35% or less, left ventricular end-diastolic dimension of at least 55 mm, QRS duration longer than 130 milliseconds, and a stable heart failure medical regimen for at least 1 month. Primary end points were the 6-minute hall walk, quality of life, and NYHA class. Improvement was shown for all three primary end points: quality of life, as determined by the "Minnesota Living With Heart Failure Questionnaire" (a 9-unit improvement, $P=0.003$); NYHA functional class (one class improvement,

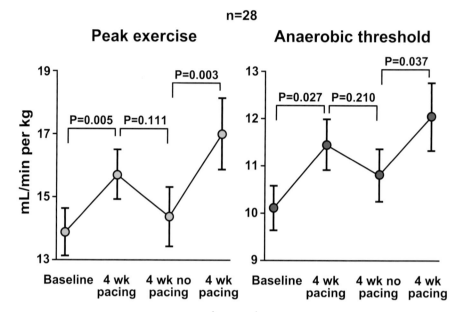

Figure 14. Changes achieved in peak $\dot{V}O_2$ and $\dot{V}O_2$ anaerobic threshold in the PATH-CHF trial. The values deteriorated when pacing was turned "off." (Data from Auricchio A, Stellbrink C, Butter C, Sack S, Vogt J, Misier AR, et al. Clinical efficacy of cardiac resynchronization therapy using left ventricular pacing in heart failure patients stratified by severity of ventricular conduction delay. J Am Coll Cardiol 2003;42:2109-16.)

Table 4. Comparison of End Points at 12 and 24 Months of 67 Patients in Normal Sinus Rhythm and NYHA Functional Class III

End point	Baseline	12 months	24 months
Heart rate, beats/min	75±12	70±10*	70±13*
Six-minute hall walk, m	340±97	418±112*	386±150*
Peak $\dot{V}O_2$, mL/kg per min	14±4.5	16.6±3.6*	NA
Quality-of-life score	45±23	30±22*	29±22*
NYHA functional class	2.8±0.4	2.1±0.5*	2.1±0.6*
LVEF	24±7.7	30±12*	NA

LVEF, left ventricular ejection fraction; NA, not available; NYHA, New York Heart Association.
*$P<0.01$ compared with baseline.

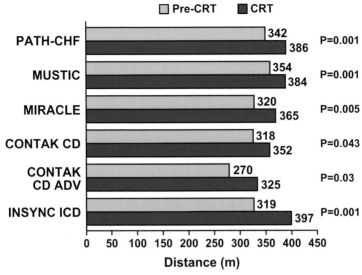

Figure 15. Change in 6-minute hall walk in five cardiac resynchronization therapy (CRT) studies. All the studies consistently demonstrated improvement in this variable, as noted by the *P* value for each study. CONTAK CD ADV (Advanced) represents the patients enrolled in the CONTAK CD trial who were in New York Heart Association class III or IV. CONTAK CD represents all the patients enrolled in the trial.

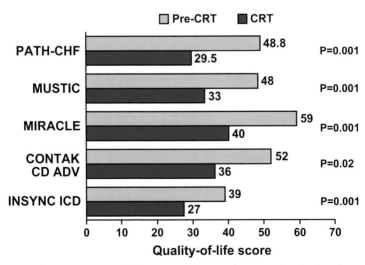

Figure 16. Change in quality-of-life scores in five cardiac resynchronization therapy (CRT) studies. All the studies consistently demonstrated improvement in the score, as noted by the *P* value for each study. CONTAK CD ADV (Advanced) represents the patients enrolled in the CONTAK CD trial who were in New York Heart Association class III or IV.

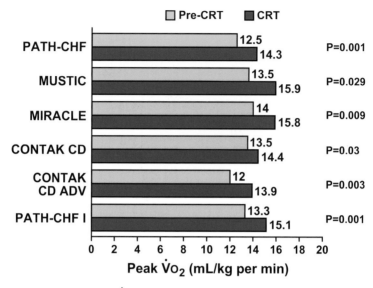

Figure 17. Change in peak $\dot{V}O_2$ in five cardiac resynchronization therapy (CRT) studies. All consistently demonstrated improvement in peak $\dot{V}O_2$. All but one study (MIRACLE) met statistical significance as noted by *P* values. CONTAK CD ADV (Advanced) represents the patients enrolled in the CONTAK CD trial who were in New York Heart Association class III or IV. CONTAK CD represents all the patients enrolled in the trial.

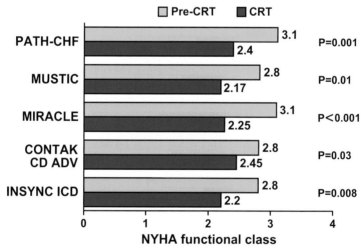

Figure 18. Change in New York Heart Association (NYHA) functional class in five cardiac resynchronization therapy (CRT) studies. All consistently demonstrated improvement in functional class. CONTAK CD ADV (Advanced) represents patients enrolled in the CONTAK CD trial who were in NYHA class III or IV.

P<0.001), and the 6-minute hall walk (a 30-meter improvement, P=0.003). The individual primary end points and various combinations of end points in the InSync study are summarized in Table 5.

MIRACLE demonstrated improvement in the secondary end points of peak oxygen consumption (P=0.009) and total exercise time (P=0.001). In addition, LVEF increased and left ventricular end-diastolic dimension, area of the mitral regurgitant jet, and duration of the QRS interval all decreased in the group that had resynchronization "on" (all P<0.001).

The Ventak-CHF/CONTAK CD study was a randomized, controlled, double-blind study that compared active cardiac resynchronization therapy with no pacing.[51] (Initially, it had a 3-month crossover trial design but later was changed to a 6-month parallel control study design.) Even though CONTAK CD includes defibrillation, the results of the trial are pertinent to a pure "resynchronization" discussion and are included here as well as in a subsequent chapter. The patients enrolled in the study had NYHA functional class II-IV heart failure, LVEF of 35% or less, QRS duration longer than 120 milliseconds, and an accepted indication for an implantable cardioverter-defibrillator (ICD). The primary end point was a composite of mortality, hospitalizations for heart failure, and episodes of ventricular tachycardia or ventricular fibrillation.

A total of 581 patients were randomly assigned: 248 into the 3-month crossover study and 333 into the 6-month parallel controlled trial.[35] The primary composite end point did not reach statistical significance favoring the resynchronization group. Secondary end points, including peak $\dot{V}O_2$, 6-minute hall walk distance, quality-of-life

---

Table 5. Improvement in End Points of InSync Study

End point	Improvement, % of patients		P value
	Control	Treatment	
Primary end points met			
NYHA functional class	37.9	67.6	<0.001
QOL score	44.0	57.6	0.017
Six-minute hall walk	27.1	45.4	<0.001
More than 1 end point met			
Hall walk & QOL score	18.1	32.6	0.003
Hall walk & NYHA class	14.8	37.6	<0.001
QOL score & NYHA class	25.9	47.1	<0.001
All 3 end points	12.0	29.7	<0.001

NYHA, New York Heart Association; QOL, quality of life.

score, and NYHA class were significantly improved in the group with resynchronization compared with inactive control subjects. When NYHA class III or IV patients were analyzed separately (i.e., class II patients were excluded), the improvement in these end points was even more significant. Also, left ventricular end-systolic and end-diastolic dimensions were decreased.

The InSync III trial used inclusion criteria and follow-up identical to those of MIRACLE. The purpose of this trial was to demonstrate the safety and efficacy of programmable VV timing or sequential biventricular timing. This trial design was the same as for MIRACLE. A total of 264 patients were enrolled, and the trial prospectively analyzed the incremental benefit of variable VV timing on the 6-minute hall walk, NYHA functional class, and quality-of-life score.

Sequential biventricular pacing improved the echocardiographic variable of aortic velocity time integral (VTI) by 11.2% at 3 months. When this group was compared with the 3-month data of the MIRACLE control group, all three end points assessed in the InSync III group demonstrated statistically significant improvement.[52]

The COMPANION trial compared optimized pharmacologic therapy (OPT) to CRT with OPT vs. CRT-D with OPT. Results from this study are discussed in Chapter 7.

Other controlled studies of CRT are ongoing. Cardiac Resynchronization in Heart Failure (CARE-HF) is a multicenter prospective, randomized controlled trial comparing optimal medical therapy only and CRT with optimal medical therapy.[53] Approximately 800 patients were enrolled in the study, which is now in the follow-up phase, with results expected in 2004.

Other trials that assessed combined CRT and defibrillation are discussed in Chapter 7.

Patients With Chronic Atrial Fibrillation

Fewer data are available about CRT in patients with atrial fibrillation than in patients with normal sinus rhythm. Several reports merit discussion. Some of these are uncontrolled studies,[30,54-56] and others are controlled but involve only a small number of patients.[57-59]

Studies that compared patients with atrial fibrillation with those in normal sinus rhythm found no significant difference between the measured variables, suggesting that patients with atrial fibrillation and those with normal sinus rhythm derive similar benefit from CRT[57-59] (Table 6).

MUSTIC-Atrial Fibrillation enrolled 65 patients with chronic atrial fibrillation and 48 were randomly assigned to CRT or no CRT. The study design was the same as described for MUSTIC-Sinus Rhythm. Similar to the normal sinus rhythm group, the atrial fibrillation group had significant improvement in the quality-of-life score, $\dot{V}O_2$, NYHA functional class, and 6-minute hall walk. These improvements were sustained at 12 and 24 months (Table 7).

Table 6. Trials of Cardiac Resynchronization Therapy in Patients With Atrial Fibrillation

Study/author	Type of study	No. of patients	Results
Leclercq	Observational	15 in AF *vs.* 22 in NSR	Mortality higher in AF group Symptoms improved in both groups with mean 35% decrease in NYHA score Increase in $\dot{V}O_2$ was significant in both but greater in AF group
Etienne	Observational	11 in AF *vs.* 17 in NSR	Comparable hemodynamic benefits for both groups with both LV & BiV pacing
Italian InSync Registry	Observational	25 in AF *vs.* 126 in NSR	Similar & significant improvements for NSR and AF groups in QRS duration, LVEF, NYHA class change, QOL, 6-min hall walk
MUSTIC-AF	Randomized controlled	65 enrolled, 48 randomized	Exercise tolerance & QOL improved Significant increase in LVEF Decreased hospitalizations for CHF Benefits of BiV pacing sustained for AF group
PAVE (left ventricular-based stimulation Post AV nodal ablation evaluation)	Randomized controlled	Study ongoing, target enrollment of 600	Primary end points: Functional ability by distance during 6-min hall walk QOL measured by score of SF-36 Electrical performance of the lead Overall adverse event rate in RV, LV and BiV groups Lead-related adverse event rate Rate of successful implantation of the lead

AF, atrial fibrillation; BiV, biventricular; LV, left ventricular; LVEF, left ventricular ejection fraction; NSR, normal sinus rhythm; NYHA, New York Heart Association; QOL, quality-of-life score; RV, right ventricular.

Table 7. Effect of Cardiac Resynchronization Therapy at 12 and 24 Months in Patients With Chronic Atrial Fibrillation

Variable	Baseline	12 months	24 months
Heart rate, beats/min	75±15	76±7	71±12
Six-minute hall walk, m	325±82	370±87*	362±99*
Peak V̇O$_2$, mL/kg per min	13±4	14±3.5	NA
Quality-of-life score	45±23	31±17*	32±20*
NYHA class	3±0	2.2±0.5*	2.2±0.5*
LVEF, %	26±7.7	30±8*	NA

LVEF, left ventricular ejection fraction; NA, not available; NYHA, New York Heart Association.
*$P<0.01$ compared with baseline.

Clinical Implications of the Data

Although the application of CRT is still in its infancy, some clinical guidelines can be suggested on the basis of the available data. CRT should be considered only for patients who remain symptomatic despite a stable and optimized medical regimen. Unless the medical regimen is not tolerated, it should include the following: an angiotensin-converting enzyme inhibitor or angiotensin receptor blocker, a β-blocker, spironolactone, a diuretic, and digoxin. The use of these agents and other strategies to prevent the development of heart failure are discussed in Chapter 1.

CRT should not be considered an alternative to medical therapy. As pointed out in Chapter 1, many patients with congestive heart failure do not receive an optimized medical program. Physicians who are considering referring a patient for CRT or contemplating implantation of a CRT device should first be rigorous in optimizing the medical regimen.

Implantation criteria as labeled by the U.S. Food and Drug Administration (FDA) are as follows:
- Stable and optimized medical regimen
- NYHA functional class III or IV
- QRS duration ≥120 to 130 milliseconds*
- LVEF ≤35%

Currently, CRT is approved for patients in NYHA functional class III or IV. Sufficient data are not available to argue for CRT in patients in NYHA functional class II. Studies to assess the long-term effect of CRT or left ventricular pacing in

*FDA labeling includes a variation in QRS width required due to specific manufacturers' clinical trials and QRS width required for inclusion in the clinical trial.

patients with LBBB or nonspecific intraventricular conduction defect and normal or near-normal left ventricular function have been designed but not implemented. If CRT results in reverse remodeling in patients with severe left ventricular dysfunction, might it not prevent remodeling if initiated early in the course of a cardiomyopathic process? Also, should pacing for standard pacing indications be left ventricular pacing instead of the traditional right ventricular apical pacing when coronary sinus lead technology and implant techniques, speed, and complication rates are similar to those of right ventricular endocardial leads? No data exist, but studies undoubtedly will be performed to answer this question.

None of the CRT trials described above were designed as "mortality" trials. However, the effect of CRT on mortality and hospitalization has been assessed in a meta-analysis of the CONTAK-CD, InSync ICD, MIRACLE, and MUSTIC trials.[60] In this analysis, CRT decreased death from progressive congestive heart failure by 51% compared with controls (Fig. 19) and reduced hospitalizations for congestive heart failure by 29% (Fig. 20).

The data on CRT in atrial fibrillation are summarized above and, although the data are limited, we think that many of these patients will benefit from CRT.

As discussed in the section on "Mechanisms," the appropriateness of the current criterion for QRS duration is questionable. With the information available about left ventricular interventricular dyssynchrony in patients with normal surface QRS, the use of surface QRS as a selection criterion must be reconsidered.

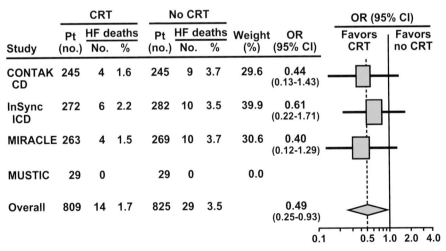

Figure 19. Meta-analysis of death from progressive heart failure (HF) in patients randomly assigned to cardiac resynchronization therapy (CRT) vs. no CRT. CI, confidence interval; OR, odds ratio; Pt, patient. (From Bradley et al.[60] By permission of the American Medical Association.)

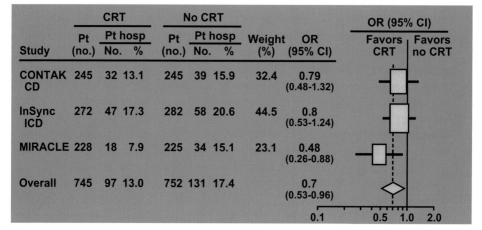

Study	CRT Pt (no.)	Pt hosp No.	Pt hosp %	No CRT Pt (no.)	Pt hosp No.	Pt hosp %	Weight (%)	OR (95% CI)	OR (95% CI) Favors CRT	Favors no CRT
CONTAK CD	245	32	13.1	245	39	15.9	32.4	0.79 (0.48-1.32)		
InSync ICD	272	47	17.3	282	58	20.6	44.5	0.8 (0.53-1.24)		
MIRACLE	228	18	7.9	225	34	15.1	23.1	0.48 (0.26-0.88)		
Overall	745	97	13.0	752	131	17.4		0.7 (0.53-0.96)		

Figure 20. Meta-analysis of hospitalization for heart failure in patients randomized to cardiac resynchronization therapy (CRT) vs. no CRT. CI, confidence interval; hosp, hospitalized; OR, odds ratio; Pt, patient. (From Bradley et al.[60] By permission of the American Medical Association.)

Another subset of patients who may be considered for CRT are those who have a pacemaker but have an underlying intrinsic narrow QRS. If the patient has pacing for the majority of the time, right ventricular pacing-induced left ventricular dyssynchrony occurs. CRT may normalize left ventricular activation, as noted above. In fact, recent information suggests that patients with pacing not only benefit from CRT but may benefit more than patients who have an intrinsic conduction delay, because of the potentially greater adverse effects of stimulating from the right ventricular apex.[59]

Similarly, the absolute degree of left ventricular systolic dysfunction (i.e., the absolute value for LVEF) has not been established. Studies have largely included patients with an LVEF of 35% or less. Some pharmacologic heart failure studies suggest that this perhaps should be liberalized to 40% or less.

In addition to satisfying the clinical criteria discussed here, the patient should be given certain basic information before referral. Although it is important for the patient to be optimistic about the potential improvement from CRT, caregivers must provide realistic information. It is too early in the CRT experience to know which patient will have a positive response to this treatment. Patients should understand that although rigorous studies have demonstrated marked improvement in some patients, not every patient will have a response to CRT.

Summary

LBBB has detrimental effects on left ventricular performance and is a predictor of mortality of patients with severe left ventricular dysfunction. The effects of LBBB on systolic and diastolic left ventricular function may induce or exacerbate the remodeling process that characterizes the progression of left ventricular dysfunction and the symptoms of congestive heart failure. Left ventricular or biventricular pacing seems to restore the homogeneity of left ventricular contraction and the mechanical synchrony between left and right ventricular systole. This is associated with improved systolic myocardial function acutely and long-term improvement in the clinical status of patients with severe congestive heart failure and LBBB. Currently, it appears that the longer the QRS duration and the more dyssynchronous the ventricular contraction, the more likely that pacing will improve left ventricular function. In some patients, left ventricular pacing only is hemodynamically equivalent or superior to biventricular pacing. Because some degree of delay between left and right ventricular mechanical activation seems desirable, biventricular pacing systems that allow independent stimulation of the right and left ventricles are being evaluated. Careful and individualized selection of the pacing site and variables appears necessary to optimize the hemodynamic benefits for a patient.

Because of the high incidence of sudden cardiac death in patients with severe congestive heart failure, the combination of biventricular pacing with ICD therapy will likely provide additional benefit, as discussed in the section on ICD therapy in congestive heart failure.

References

1. Hochleitner M, Hortnagl H, Ng CK, Gschnitzer F, Zechmann W. Usefulness of physiologic dual-chamber pacing in drug-resistant idiopathic dilated cardiomyopathy. Am J Cardiol 1990;66:198-202.

2. Hochleitner M, Hortnagl H, Fridrich L, Gschnitzer F. Long-term efficacy of physiologic dual-chamber pacing in the treatment of end-stage idiopathic dilated cardiomyopathy. Am J Cardiol 1992;70:1320-5.

3. Brecker SJ, Xiao HB, Sparrow J, Gibson DG. Effects of dual-chamber pacing with short atrioventricular delay in dilated cardiomyopathy. Lancet 1992;340:1308-12.

4. Gold MR, Feliciano Z, Gottlieb SS, Fisher ML. Dual-chamber pacing with a short atrioventricular delay in congestive heart failure: a randomized study. J Am Coll Cardiol 1995;26:967-73.

5. Linde C, Gadler F, Edner M, Nordlander R, Rosenqvist M, Ryden L. Results of atrioventricular synchronous pacing with optimized delay in patients with severe congestive heart failure. Am J Cardiol 1995;75:919-23.

6. Innes D, Leitch JW, Fletcher PJ. VDD pacing at short atrioventricular intervals does not improve cardiac output in patients with dilated heart failure. Pacing Clin Electrophysiol 1994;17:959-65.

7. Nishimura RA, Hayes DL, Holmes DR Jr, Tajik AJ. Mechanism of hemodynamic improvement by dual-chamber pacing for severe left ventricular dysfunction: an acute Doppler and catheterization hemodynamic study. J Am Coll Cardiol 1995;25:281-8.

8. Gregoratos G, Cheitlin MD, Conill A, Epstein AE, Fellows C, Ferguson TB Jr, et al. ACC/AHA guidelines for implantation of cardiac pacemakers and antiarrhythmia devices: a report of the American College of Cardiology/American Heart Association Task Force on Practice Guidelines (Committee on Pacemaker Implantation). J Am Coll Cardiol 1998;31:1175-209.

9. Shamin W, Francis DP, Yousufuddin M, Anker S, Coats AJS. Intraventricular conduction delay: a predictor of mortality in chronic heart failure? [Abstract.] Eur Heart J 1989;19:147.

10. Lamp B, Hammel D, Kerber S, Deng M, Breithardt G, Block M. Multisite pacing in severe heart failure: how many patients are eligible? [Abstract.] Pacing Clin Electrophysiol 1998;24:973.

11. Aaronson KD, Schwartz JS, Chen TM, Wong KL, Goin JE, Mancini DM. Development and prospective validation of a clinical index to predict survival in ambulatory patients referred for cardiac transplant evaluation. Circulation 1997;95:2660-7.

12. Schoeller R, Andresen D, Buttner P, Oezcelik K, Vey G, Schroder R. First- or second-degree atrioventricular block as a risk factor in idiopathic dilated cardiomyopathy. Am J Cardiol 1993;71:720-6.

13. Gottipaty VK, Krelis SP, Lu F, Spencer EP, Shusterman V, Weiss R, et al., for the VEST Investigators. The resting electrocardiogram provides a sensitive and inexpensive marker of prognosis in patients with chronic congestive heart failure (abstract). J Am Coll Cardiol 1999;33:145A.

14. Wilensky RL, Yudelman P, Cohen AI, Fletcher RD, Atkinson J, Virmani R, et al. Serial electrocardiographic changes in idiopathic dilated cardiomyopathy confirmed at necropsy. Am J Cardiol 1988;62:276-83.

15. Grines CL, Bashore TM, Boudoulas H, Olson S, Shafer P, Wooley CF. Functional abnormalities in isolated left bundle branch block: the effect of interventricular asynchrony. Circulation 1989;79:845-53.

16. Gerber TC, Nishimura RA, Holmes DR Jr, Lloyd MA, Zehr KJ, Tajik AJ, et al. Left ventricular and biventricular pacing in congestive heart failure. Mayo Clin Proc 2001;76:803-12.

17. Wyndham CR, Meeran MK, Smith T, Saxena A, Engelman RM, Levitsky S, et al. Epicardial activation of the intact human heart without conduction defect. Circulation 1979;59:161-8.

18. Wyndham CR, Smith T, Meeran MK, Mammana R, Levitsky S, Rosen KM. Epicardial activation in patients with left bundle branch block. Circulation 1980;61:696-703.

19. Bramlet DA, Morris KG, Coleman RE, Albert D, Cobb FR. Effect of rate-dependent left bundle branch block on global and regional left ventricular function. Circulation 1983;67:1059-65.

20. Garrigue S, Reuter S, Labeque JN, Jais P, Hocini M, Shah DC, et al. Usefulness of biventricular pacing in patients with congestive heart failure and right bundle branch block. Am J Cardiol 2001;88:1436-41.

21. Kass DA, Chen CH, Curry C, Talbot M, Berger R, Fetics B, et al. Improved left ventricular mechanics from acute VDD pacing in patients with dilated cardiomyopathy and ventricular conduction delay. Circulation 1999;99:1567-73.

22. Auricchio A, Klein H, Tockman B, Sack S, Stellbrink C, Neuzner J, et al. Transvenous biventricular pacing for heart failure: can the obstacles be overcome? Am J Cardiol 1999;83:136D-42D.

23. Saxon LA, Kerwin WF, Cahalan MK, Kalman JM, Olgin JE, Foster E, et al. Acute effects of intraoperative multisite ventricular pacing on left ventricular function and activation/contraction sequence in patients with depressed ventricular function. J Cardiovasc Electrophysiol 1998;9:13-21.

24. Søgaard P, Egeblad H, Kim WY, Jensen HK, Pedersen AK, Kristensen BØ, et al. Tissue Doppler imaging predicts improved systolic performance and reversed left ventricular remodeling during long-term cardiac resynchronization therapy. J Am Coll Cardiol 2002;40:723-30.

25. Yu CM, Lin H, Zhang Q, Sanderson JE. High prevalence of left ventricular systolic and diastolic asynchrony in patients with congestive heart failure and normal QRS duration. Heart 2003;89:54-60.

26. Bax JJ, Molhoek SG, van Erven L, Voogd PJ, Somer S, Boersma E, et al. Usefulness of myocardial tissue Doppler echocardiography to evaluate left ventricular dyssynchrony before and after biventricular pacing in patients with idiopathic dilated cardiomyopathy. Am J Cardiol 2003;91:94-7.

27. Lee TH, Hamilton MA, Stevenson LW, Moriguchi JD, Fonarow GC, Child JS, et al. Impact of left ventricular cavity size on survival in advanced heart failure. Am J Cardiol 1993;72:672-6.

28. Abraham WT, Fisher WG, Smith AL, Delurgio DB, Leon AR, Loh E, et al., for the MIRACLE Study Group. Cardiac resynchronization in chronic heart failure. N Engl J Med 2002;346:1845-53.

29. Yu CM, Chau E, Sanderson JE, Fan K, Tang MO, Fung WH, et al. Tissue Doppler echocardiographic evidence of reverse remodeling and improved synchronicity by simultaneously delaying regional contraction after biventricular pacing therapy in heart failure. Circulation 2002;105:438-45.

30. Etienne Y, Mansourati J, Gilard M, Valls-Bertault V, Boschat J, Benditt DG, et al. Evaluation of left ventricular based pacing in patients with congestive heart failure and atrial fibrillation. Am J Cardiol 1999;83:1138-40.

31. Kim WY, Søgaard P, Mortensen PT, Jensen HK, Pedersen AK, Kristensen BØ, et al. Three dimensional echocardiography documents haemodynamic improvement by biventricular pacing in patients with severe heart failure. Heart 2001;85:514-20.

32. St. John Sutton MG, Plappert T, Abraham WT, Smith AL, DeLurgio DB, Leon AR, et al., for the Multicenter InSync Randomized Clinical Evaluation (MIRACLE) Study Group. Effect of cardiac resynchronization therapy on left ventricular size and function in chronic heart failure. Circulation 2003;107:1985-90.

33. Breithardt OA, Sinha AM, Schwammenthal E, Bidaoui N, Markus KU, Franke A, et al. Acute effects of cardiac resynchronization therapy on functional mitral regurgitation in advanced systolic heart failure [published erratum appears in J Am Coll Cardiol 2003;41:1852]. J Am Coll Cardiol 2003;41:765-70.

34. Walker S, Levy TM, Rex S, Paul VE. Biventricular pacing decreases ventricular arrhythmia [abstract]. Circulation 2000;102 Suppl 2:II-692-II-3.

35. Francis GS, Cohn JN, Johnson G, Rector TS, Goldman S, Simon A, for The V-HeFT VA Cooperative Studies Group. Plasma norepinephrine, plasma renin activity, and congestive heart failure: relations to survival and the effects of therapy in V-HeFT II. Circulation 1993;87 Suppl:VI-40-8.

36. Saxon LA, DeMarco T, Chatterjee K, Kerwin WF, Boehmer J, for the Vigor and Ventak-CHF Investigators. Chronic biventricular pacing decreases serum norepinephrine in dilated heart failure patients with the greatest sympathetic activation at baseline [abstract]. Pacing Clin Electrophysiol 1999;22:830.

37. Sinha AM, Filzmaier K, Breithardt OA, Kunz D, Graf J, Markus KU, et al. Usefulness of brain natriuretic peptide release as a surrogate marker of the efficacy of long-term cardiac resynchronization therapy in patients with heart failure. Am J Cardiol 2003;91:755-8.

38. Bocker D, Block M, Auricchio A, Stellbrink C, Carlson G, Zhu C, et al. Resynchronization may restore autonomic balance in heart failure. Europace 2001:2 Suppl:B87.

39. Nolan J, Batin PD, Andrews R, Lindsay SJ, Brooksby P, Mullen M, et al. Prospective study of heart rate variability and mortality in chronic heart failure: results of the United Kingdom Heart Failure Evaluation and Assessment of Risk Trial (UK-HEART). Circulation 1998;98:1510-6.

40. Cazeau S, Ritter P, Bakdach S, Lazarus A, Limousin M, Henao L, et al. Four chamber pacing in dilated cardiomyopathy. Pacing Clin Electrophysiol 1994;17:1974-9.

41. Foster AH, Gold MR, McLaughlin JS. Acute hemodynamic effects of atrio-biventricular pacing in humans. Ann Thorac Surg 1995;59:294-300.

42. Cazeau S, Ritter P, Lazarus A, Gras D, Backdach H, Mundler O, et al. Multisite pacing for end-stage heart failure: early experience. Pacing Clin Electrophysiol 1996;19:1748-57.

43. Blanc JJ, Etienne Y, Gilard M, Mansourati J, Munier S, Boschat J, et al. Evaluation of different ventricular pacing sites in patients with severe heart failure: results of an acute hemodynamic study. Circulation 1997;96:3273-7.

44. Gras D, Mabo P, Tang T, Luttikuis O, Chatoor R, Pedersen AK, et al. Multisite pacing as a supplemental treatment of congestive heart failure: preliminary results of the Medtronic Inc. InSync Study. Pacing Clin Electrophysiol 1998;21:2249-55.

45. Leclercq C, Cazeau S, Le Breton H, Ritter P, Mabo P, Gras D, et al. Acute hemodynamic effects of biventricular DDD pacing in patients with end-stage heart failure. J Am Coll Cardiol 1998;32:1825-31.

46. Gras D, Leclercq C, Tang AS, Bucknall C, Luttikhuis HO, Kirstein-Pedersen A. Cardiac resynchronization therapy in advanced heart failure the multicenter InSync clinical study. Eur J Heart Fail 2002;4:311-20.

47. Young JB, Abraham WT, Smith AL, Leon AR, Lieberman R, Wilkoff B, et al., for the Multicenter InSync ICD Randomized Clinical Evaluation (MIRACLE ICD) Trial Investigators. Combined cardiac resynchronization and implantable cardioversion defibrillation in advanced chronic heart failure: the MIRACLE ICD Trial. JAMA 2003;289:2685-94.
48. Auricchio A, Stellbrink C, Sack S, Block M, Vogt J, Bakker P, et al. The Pacing Therapies for Congestive Heart Failure (PATH-CHF) study: rationale, design, and endpoints of a prospective randomized multicenter study. Am J Cardiol 1999;83:130D-5D
49. O'Cochlain B, Delurgio D, Leon A, Langberg J. The effect of variation in the interval between right and left ventricular activation on paced QRS duration. Pacing Clin Electrophysiol 2001;24:1780-2.
50. Cazeau S, Leclercq C, Lavergne T, Walker S, Varma C, Linde C, et al., for the Multisite Stimulation in Cardiomyopathies (MUSTIC) Study Investigators. Effects of multisite biventricular pacing in patients with heart failure and intraventricular conduction delay. N Engl J Med 2001;344:873-80.
51. Thackray S, Coletta A, Jones P, Dunn A, Clark AL, Cleland JG. Clinical trials update: highlights of the Scientific Sessions of Heart Failure 2001, a meeting of the Working Group on Heart Failure of the European Society of Cardiology. CONTAK-CD, CHRISTMAS, OPTIME-CHF. Eur J Heart Fail 2001;3:491-4.
52. The US InSync III Trial. Effect of cardiac resynchronization therapy with sequential biventricular pacing on Doppler-derived left ventricular stroke volume, functional status and exercise capacity in patients with ventricular dysfunction and conduction delay [abstract]. Pacing Clin Electrophysiol 2002;24:558.
53. Cleland JG, Daubert JC, Erdmann E, Freemantle N, Gras D, Kappenberger L, et al., CARE-HF study Steering Committee and Investigators. The CARE-HF study (CArdiac REsynchronisation in Heart Failure study): rationale, design and end-points. Eur J Heart Fail 2001;3:481-9.
54. Leclercq C, Victor F, Alonso C, Pavin D, Revault D'Allones G, Bansard JY, et al. Comparative effects of permanent biventricular pacing for refractory heart failure in patients with stable sinus rhythm or chronic atrial fibrillation. Am J Cardiol 2000;85:1154-6.
55. Zardini M, Tritto M, Bargiggia G, Forzani T, Santini M, Perego GB, et al., the InSync Italian Registry Investigators. The InSync Italian Registry: analysis of clinical outcome and considerations on the selection of candidates to left ventricular resynchronization. Eur Heart J 2000;2 Suppl J:J16-J22.
56. Walker S, Levy TM, Coats AJ, Peters NS, Paul VE, for the Imperial College Cardiac Electrophysiology Group. Bi-ventricular pacing in congestive cardiac failure: current experience and future directions. Eur Heart J 2000;21:884-9.
57. Leclercq C, Walker S, Linde C, Clementy J, Marshall AJ, Ritter P, et al. Comparative effects of permanent biventricular and right-univentricular pacing in heart failure patients with chronic atrial fibrillation. Eur Heart J 2002;23:1780-7.
58. Garrigue S, Bordachar P, Reuter S, Jais P, Kobeissi A, Gaggini G, et al. Comparison of permanent left ventricular and biventricular pacing in patients with heart failure and chronic atrial fibrillation: prospective haemodynamic study. Heart 2002;87:529-34.
59. Leon AR, Greenberg JM, Kanuru N, Baker CM, Mera FV, Smith AL, et al. Cardiac resynchronization in patients with congestive heart failure and chronic atrial fibrillation: effect of upgrading to biventricular pacing after chronic right ventricular pacing. J Am Coll Cardiol 2002;39:1258-63.
60. Bradley DJ, Bradley EA, Baughman KL, Berger RD, Calkins H, Goodman SN, et al. Cardiac resynchronization and death from progressive heart failure: a meta-analysis of randomized controlled trials. JAMA 2003;289:730-40.

CHAPTER 3

Electrocardiogram Interpretation With Biventricular Pacing Devices

Samuel J. Asirvatham, MD

Introduction

With the increasing use of and requirement for familiarity with biventricular pacing systems, several key questions are often asked[1-3]: Is the left ventricular lead capturing the ventricle? Has the left ventricular lead moved from its initial position at implantation? What is the degree of fusion of ventricular activation between the left and right ventricular pacing leads?[4] Although a complete answer to these questions requires thorough analysis of the chest radiograph, electrocardiogram (ECG), and device interrogation, the ECG often provides immediate and reliable answers to these questions.[5,6] This chapter outlines the ECG vector principles that underlie the ability to answer these questions and then discusses the characteristic ECG signature sites for right ventricular and various left ventricular lead positions. Next, the chapter presents an approach to analyzing a biventricular-paced ECG to ascertain the extent and site of the pacing lead capture as well as the relative contribution of the two leads.[7] Finally, the chapter includes a few examples of typical ECGs and a demonstration of applying the methods.

Principles of Electrocardiographic and Vector-Cardiographic Interpretation Relevant to Biventricular Devices

The fundamental principles for interpreting biventricular device ECGs are as follows: 1) ECG leads generally represent widely spaced bipoles.[8,9] The positive pole or equivalent for each standard frontal or chest lead is presented diagrammatically. 2) Whenever a depolarization front, that is, cardiac activation, proceeds toward a positive pole of an ECG lead, a positive deflection is inscribed. It follows that a negative deflection in a given ECG lead suggests electrical activation proceeding away from the positive electrode of that lead.[10,11]

On the basis of knowing the configuration of a given lead and understanding the significance of a positive or negative deflection, the vector of activation can easily be estimated. Therefore, a positive R wave in lead I suggests electrical activation proceeding from the right side of the ventricle to the left, because the positive electrode for lead I is located on the left arm. This leftward vector may represent activation from the right ventricle toward the left ventricle or from the interventricular septum to the free wall of the left ventricle.[8,9] The principles for this type of analysis with biventricular devices are exactly those used to identify the site of earliest activation in Wolff-Parkinson-White syndrome and ventricular tachycardia.

Left and Lateral Leads (Fig. 1)

The positive electrode or equivalent for leads I, aVL, V_5, and V_6 are all located on the left side of the body. Therefore, a positive deflection in these leads suggests activation proceeding from right to left, and conversely, a negative deflection suggests activation proceeding away from the left and lateral portions of the ventricle. However, there are important differences in the information provided within this set

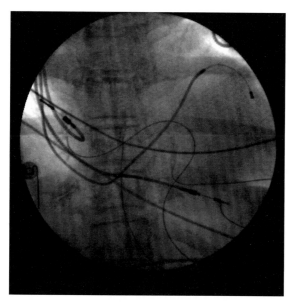

Figure 1. Pacemaker leads in the right atrial appendage and right ventricular apex are positioned in the usual fashion. The left ventricular lead courses through the coronary sinus and is placed in a lateral cardiac vein midway between the base and apex. Pacing from this left ventricular stimulation site will result in a vector that moves away from lead I and aVL and toward leads V_1 and aVR.

of leads. Lead aVL, in addition to having its positive electrode equivalent on the left side, is also superior compared with lead I. Therefore, a high superior septal site of activation that proceeds away from lead aVL toward the left lateral wall produces a negative deflection in aVL and yet is positive in lead I. The situation is similar for leads V_5 and V_6. Although their positive electrode is located on the left side of the body, it represents a relatively more inferior and apical position than the positive electrode of lead I. Therefore, an apical origin of activation may be sharply negative in V_6 but positive in lead aVL or lead I. Thus, a quick look at this set of leads will show that activation is proceeding from right to left or vice versa.[8,9]

A closer look at differences in the information or degree of positivity and negativity between these leads gives additional information about a superior or inferior leftward location. Right ventricular pacing from the apex always produces a positive deflection in leads I and aVL and is variably positive in leads V_5 and V_6. In comparison, typical left ventricular pacing from a lateral cardiac vein (see below) produces a sharp negative deflection (S wave) in lead I. Whether leads aVL and V_5 and V_6 are also negative depends on whether the lead is located more basally (negative in aVL) or apically (negative in V_5 and V_6).

Inferior Leads

Leads II, III, and aVF have their positive electrode or equivalent located inferiorly (near the feet). Therefore, a positive deflection in these leads suggests activation proceeding from a superior location toward the feet. Conversely, activation from an inferior site in the ventricle produces an S wave or negative deflection in these leads.[12] There are some important differences in the information conveyed within this group of leads. The orientation of lead III is such that the positive electrode, although inferior, is relatively more rightward than lead II. Therefore, right ventricular pacing from an inferior location is relatively more negative in lead III than in lead II. Conversely, pacing from a left ventricular inferior site such as the middle cardiac vein is negative in both leads II and III; however, it is relatively more negative in lead II than in lead III. Thus, the degree of negativity (i.e., depth of the S wave) compared between leads II and III will clarify further whether an inferior pacing site is rightward or leftward on the inferior portion of the heart.

Rightward Chest Leads—Leads V_1, aVR, and III

These leads have their positive electrode or equivalent located on the right side of the body.[13] Therefore, a negative deflection in these leads suggests activation proceeding from a right-sided stimulation site toward the left and vice versa. There are important differences in the information provided within this set of leads. Although lead V_1 represents a rightward positive electrode, it is placed on the anterior chest. Therefore, lead V_1 is negative either with a right-sided stimulation site or an anterior stimulation site. Conversely, pacing from the left side or a posterior site produces a positive deflection (right bundle branch block pattern) in lead V_1. Because the left ventricle is posterior and to the left of the right ventricle, most left ventricular pacing sites produce a positive deflection in lead V_1 (right bundle branch block).[5] Most stimulation sites in the right ventricle are rightward and anterior to the left ventricle and, thus, produce a negative deflection in lead V_1 (left bundle branch block pattern). However, right ventricular leads placed in the right ventricular outflow tract, particularly in more leftward locations, produce a right bundle branch block pattern because the right ventricular outflow tract is located on the left side of the body compared with the left ventricular outflow tract, which is posterior and more to the right side of the body. Similarly, a lead located deep in the right ventricular apex, especially with clockwise rotated hearts, may produce a positive deflection in lead V_1.

Lead aVR, with the location of its right anterior positive electrode equivalent to lead V_1, is also a superiorly located positive electrode. Therefore, inferior and apical sites produce a positive deflection in lead aVR irrespective of a rightward or leftward orientation. Also, stimulation from anterior sites such as the basal anterior interventricular vein (see below) produces a negative deflection in lead aVR (as with lead aVL) regardless of rightward or leftward orientation.

Lead III, with its positive electrode located inferiorly and relatively rightward as described above, is negative in most typical right ventricular pacing locations. Because the right ventricular apex is both inferior and rightward, sharp negative deflections are seen in lead III. However, certain right ventricular pacing sites such as the high septum or outflow tract, although still rightward, produce a positive deflection in lead III.

Chest Leads

The positive electrodes of leads V_1 through V_6 are arranged sequentially from the right second intercostal space and drape the typical apical location. Relatively more apical locations for pacing stimulation produce a negative deflection in leads V_4, V_5, and V_6, whose positive electrodes are located at the apex. Conversely, leads located more basally produce a negative deflection in lead V_1. Analyzing the transition between negativity and positivity through the chest leads gives an idea of the apical to basal location of the pacing lead. For example, a lead placed in the posterolateral vein stimulating the posterolateral region of the left ventricle produces a negative deflection in lead I, signifying its left-sided pacing site. However, this lead alone will not provide information about whether the lead is located apically in this vein or more basally. In addition, if leads V_4, V_5, and V_6 are negative, this suggests that the lead is very apical within the posterolateral vein. However, a positive deflection in these same leads suggests a more basal location within this vein.

Leads aVR and aVL

Both these leads have their positive electrode equivalent superiorly. Therefore, apical sites of stimulation produce positive deflections in both leads, and superior sites of stimulation produce negative deflections (S waves). The positive electrode for aVL is relatively more leftward; thus, the positive electrode for aVR is relatively more rightward. Consequently, a sharp deep negative S wave in lead aVR that is deeper than the S wave in lead aVL suggests a right superior pacing site.

Summary

Although at first glance it may appear complex to analyze ECGs to define the pacing site, the analysis consists of simple deductions based on the two basic principles. Understanding where the positive electrodes for the various leads are located and knowing that a pacing site near the positive electrode of a lead produces a sharp negative S wave in that lead will facilitate further analysis.

To quickly identify the pacing lead site, the ECG deflection in leads I and aVF can be considered. Lead I, if positive, suggests a right-sided or septal pacing site and if negative, a left free-wall pacing site. A positive R wave in lead aVF suggests an anterior site (anterior interventricular vein in the high septal region), whereas a negative deflection (S wave) suggests an inferior or posterior pacing site (right ventricular apex middle cardiac vein).[14] These simple generalizations with just these two leads work in most instances; however, important exceptions exist.[8,9] A more detailed analysis of typical pacing sites follows.

Right Ventricular Pacing Sites: ECG Recognition

Typical right ventricular pacing from an apical location is relatively straightforward to recognize on an ECG (Fig. 2).[15] The key features include a left bundle branch configuration (negative in lead V_1, a rightward lead), sharp deep S waves in leads II, III, and aVF (negative in the inferior leads), and a positive deflection in leads I, aVR, and aVL (positive deflection in the superior and leftward leads). Because this pacing location is the site most commonly used during implantation, it is important to memorize this pattern.[16,17] This will allow the quick recognition of variations of this pattern. It is essential to realize that not all right ventricular pacing sites produce this signature pattern. Not recognizing the variations of this pattern is a common reason for misidentifying which lead in the biventricular system is malfunctioning or failure to capture. Extreme apical locations in the right ventricle or the relatively leftward location of a pacing site in the right ventricular outflow tract produces a positive deflection or right bundle branch block. Pacing sites high on the interventricular septum or in the outflow tract produce a positive deflection in leads II, III, and aVF. The positive R wave in lead III may be misinterpreted as a left-sided pacing site.

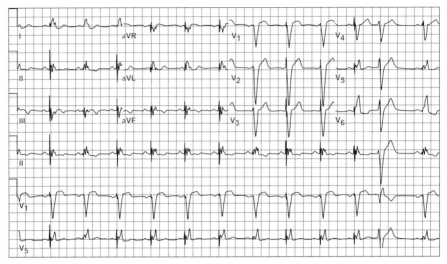

Figure 2. Pacing from the standard right ventricular position. This site is characterized by the left bundle branch block pattern in lead V_1 and positive deflections in leads I and aVL. Note that lead aVR may be negative or positive depending on how apical the lead is located. In this instance, the lead is about 1 cm proximal to the apex, as evidenced by small positive deflections in leads II and aVF.

The QRS duration is used sometimes to distinguish between a right ventricular septal pacing site and a right ventricular free-wall pacing site (Fig. 3 and 4).[18] As a generalization, septal pacing sites give rise to more narrow QRS complexes, and free-wall pacing sites are strongly positive in lead I, with wider QRS complexes. For patients who require biventricular pacing, notably those who have right and left ventricular dilation, these generalizations are unreliable. When pacing high on the interventricular septum near the base (His bundle/right bundle location), a narrow QRS with a duration less than 140 milliseconds is typical.

Left Ventricular Pacing: ECG Patterns and Their Recognition

The three main ventricular branches of the coronary sinus used for left ventricular pacing are the anterior interventricular vein, posterolateral vein, and middle cardiac vein (Fig. 5 and 6). The typical ECG signatures of pacing from these venous sites are outlined below.[19] It should be noted that most patients also have several subsidiary branches between these three main branches. Pacing from one of these other branches produces a hybrid ECG morphology that can be deduced from the patterns typical with pacing from the three main veins.

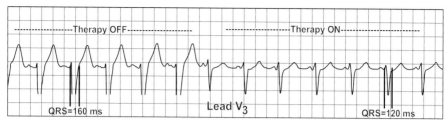

Figure 3. When biventricular stimulation therapy is turned on, the QRS duration markedly narrows. This is the anticipated result of simultaneous stimulation of the right and left ventricles. As noted in the text, stimulation from a single site on the ventricular septum may result in a narrow QRS complex. Conversely, biventricular stimulation when there is marked exit delay as well as interventricular conduction delay will not result in a narrow QRS complex despite simultaneous biventricular pacing.

Anterior Interventricular Vein

This vein runs along the left anterior descending artery in the anterior interventricular groove, and its branches follow the path of the septal and diagonal branches of the left anterior descending artery (Fig. 7-9). Typically, left lateral branches of the anterior interventricular vein interdigitate with the corresponding branches of the lateral cardiac veins. Often, the anterior interventricular vein communicates at the apex with apical tributaries of the middle cardiac vein.

Pacing from the anterior interventricular vein produces a vector that proceeds from the anterior myocardial wall toward the inferior wall. The typical ECG pattern shows a positive deflection (R wave) in leads II, III, and aVF. Lead V_1 shows a positive deflection suggestive of a right bundle branch block pattern. If one of the lateral tributaries of the anterior interventricular vein is used for pacing, then lead I will be negative and lead III will show a relatively taller R wave than lead II.[14] To distinguish whether the lead is placed relatively more apically or basally in this vein, the apical leads V_4, V_5, and V_6 as well as lead aVR can be analyzed. With apical locations in the anterior interventricular vein, leads V_4, V_5, and V_6 are typically negative and lead aVR is positive. With the more basal locations in the vein, lead aVR is negative and leads V_4, V_5, and V_6 may be positive.

Lateral and Posterolateral Cardiac Vein

The lateral and posterolateral cardiac venous tributaries follow the obtuse marginal or posterolateral coronary artery (or both). Pacing from this vein produces a negative deflection (S wave) in leads II, III, and aVF and also in lead I. This results from the posterolateral origin of the cardiac impulse and, therefore, conduction away from the posterior and inferior leads (leads II, III, and aVF) and from the lateral lead (lead I). In a more straight lateral position, lead III will be positive, as explained above, because of the relatively rightward orientation of the positive electrode in

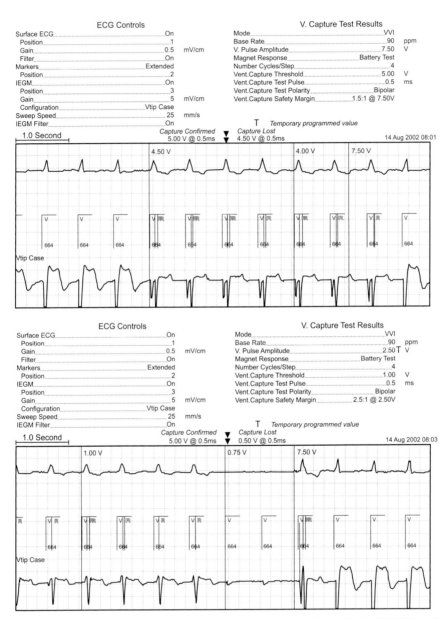

Figure 4. In this example, when the output voltage is decreased from 4 V to 3.75 V, there is intermittent loss of left ventricular lead capture. This is evidenced by the appearance of the sensed electrogram on the ventricular pacing lead. In addition, a change in QRS duration is seen intermittently. With further decrease in voltage at 0.5 V, complete loss of capture is noted. In this particular device, the presence or absence of the sensed electrogram is also useful in determining capture.

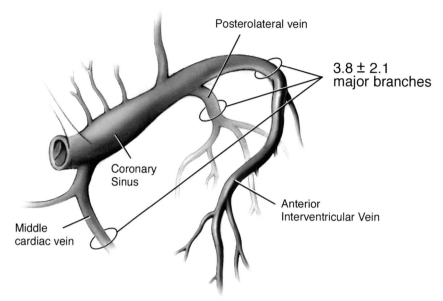

Figure 5. Typical coronary venous anatomy. Usually three to five major branches of the coronary sinus are visible at angiography and can be used for left ventricular stimulation. The three most consistent branches are the middle cardiac vein, the posterolateral or lateral vein, and the anterior interventricular vein.

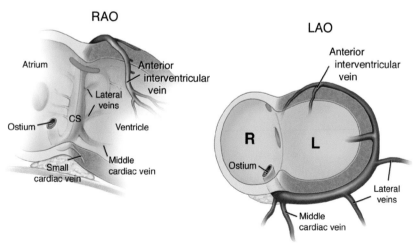

Figure 6. Typical right anterior oblique (RAO) and left anterior oblique (LAO) projections of the coronary sinus (CS) and ventricular veins. Note that the lateral veins as well as lateral branches of the anterior intraventricular vein drain the free wall of the left ventricle. Pacing from these sites results in a negative deflection in leads I and aVL.

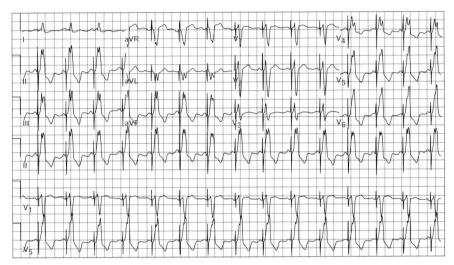

Figure 7. Biventricular, left ventricular lead in anterior vein. This electrocardiogram demonstrates features of both right and left ventricular pacing. In lead V_1, there is a small initial deflection that is positive; otherwise, the morphology appears like left bundle branch block. This suggests biventricular pacing with early activation of the left ventricle giving rise to the initial positive R wave. The left ventricular lead is likely to be in a branch of the anterior interventricular vein, as evidenced by the tall positive R waves in leads II, III, and aVF. In this example, leads I and aVL have opposite deflections. This suggests that the lead is located very basally in the anterior interventricular vein at a relatively more septal location.

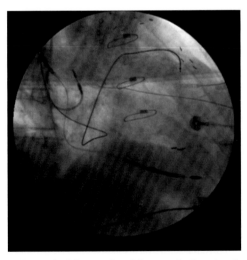

Figure 8. Fluoroscopic image in right anterior oblique projection showing the coronary sinus lead being placed in a branch of the anterior interventricular vein.

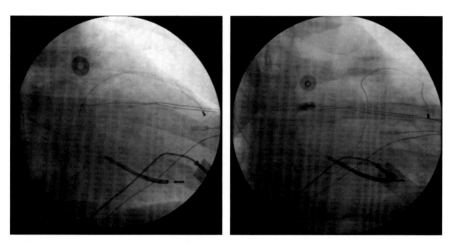

Figure 9. Right and left anterior oblique projections showing coronary sinus lead placement in the lateral branch of the anterior interventricular vein. Note that on the right anterior oblique projection it is not possible to determine whether the lead is septal or lateral. However, this is easily seen in the left anterior oblique projection.

lead III. In more posterior and septal locations, lead III will tend to be negative. Thus, although leads II and aVF for posterolateral vein pacing are almost always negative, a more septal site will also produce negativity in lead III; however, a more lateral site will produce negativity in lead I and positivity in lead III.

Middle Cardiac Vein

The middle cardiac vein runs in the posterior interventricular groove and follows the course of the posterior descending artery (Fig. 10). Tributaries to this vein drain both at the posterior right ventricle and posterior left ventricle. Distally and apically, the middle cardiac vein often communicates with apical branches of the lateral veins and the anterior interventricular vein. Pacing from this vein results in a vector that proceeds away from the inferoposterior wall of the heart. This produces a sharp negative deflection (S wave) in leads II, III, and aVF. Varying degrees of positivity in the R wave and lead V_1 that produce either a typical or atypical right bundle branch block pattern are seen. Lead I may be isoelectric or positive depending on how far septal is the branch of the middle cardiac vein from which pacing is effected. Lateral branches of the middle cardiac vein can often be used for pacing. These lateral branches may allow the lead to be passed to the lateral wall, where lead I will show a sharp negative deflection. Note that rightward branches of the middle cardiac vein often communicate with equivalent branches of the small cardiac vein. Pacing from these branches produces a left bundle branch block pattern in lead V_1 and a sharply negative deflection in lead III.

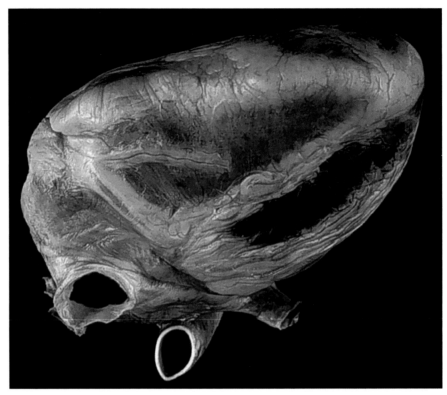

Figure 10. Autopsy specimen showing the course of the middle cardiac vein along the posterior interventricular septum. Pacing from this site results in a vector moving away from the feet. Thus, the ECG is characterized by negative deflections in leads II, III, and aVF.

Biventricular Pacing: ECG Characteristics

The ECG in biventricular pacing, with both right ventricular (RV) and left ventricular (LV) stimulation sites, represents a summated vector of the individual access of activation (RV + LV).[6] The QRS duration is typically shortened compared with stimulation at either a right ventricular or left ventricular site alone. However, this is not always true, and QRS duration alone cannot be used to determine whether stimulation is biventricular or from a single site.[20] In the follow-up of patients with biventricular pacing systems, it is often necessary to analyze the ECG to judge whether biventricular stimulation is occurring. This requires a thorough understanding of the typical ECG signatures of various left ventricular and right ventricular sites. Furthermore, when certain characteristics of the ECG suggest right ventricular apical pacing and yet others suggest left ventricular stimulation (e.g., a negative deflection in lead III and also in lead I) or a biphasic pattern in certain leads, particularly lead I (see below), two different stimulation sites are being used. The situation is more complicated when the right ventricular pacing site is not the right ventricular apex, and with certain ECGs this distinction cannot be made unless the left ventricular and right ventricular anatomical sites of stimulation are known beforehand or a previous ECG demonstrates biventricular stimulation (Fig. 11).[21]

In the following discussion, it is assumed that right ventricular pacing is from a typical apical location. If the right ventricular pacing site is elsewhere, the differences are mentioned.

Right Ventricular Apical and Anterior Interventricular Site
Lead V_1 usually shows an atypical right bundle branch pattern with an R wave preceded by either a small negative or isoelectric segment. Leads II, III, and aVF are

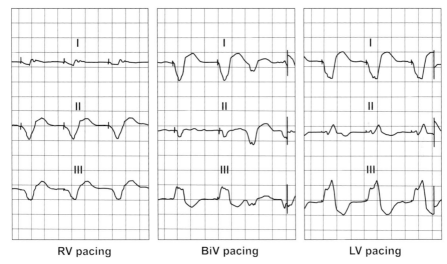

| RV pacing | BiV pacing | LV pacing |

Figure 11. Although it is ideal to have a 12-lead ECG to analyze completely biventricular (BiV) pacemaker function, often a limited number of leads are available for review. In this example, right ventricular (RV) pacing is associated with the expected negative deflections in leads II and III. However, lead I is isoelectric. Left ventricular (LV) pacing is likely from a lateral branch of the anterior inverventricular vein. Leads II and III are positive, suggesting an anterior stimulation site, and lead I is negative, suggesting a lateral stimulation site. In reviewing the BiV pacing ECG, no difference is discernible between BiV pacing and LV pacing on lead I. This is because of the minimal contribution to the vector in lead I from RV pacing. However, in analyzing lead II, a clear difference is seen. Also to be noted on this tracing is the minimal change in QRS width with BiV pacing. A clue to the reason for this lack of change can be deduced from the wide QRS also seen with the premature ventricular complex likely from the LV apex (negative lead I, negative leads II and III). With the wide QRS seen with these multiple stimulation sites, this patient likely has prominent intraventricular conduction delay.

either biphasic or isoelectric because the anterior interventricular site causes a positive deflection in these leads and right ventricular apical pacing produces a negative deflection. If either left ventricular conduction is slow or right ventricular timing is ahead of left ventricular timing[22] (see below), the inferior leads will be more typical of a right ventricular apical pacing site alone (deep S waves). Lead I will be either isoelectric or negative, suggesting an anterolateral site of stimulation from the left ventricular lead.

Right Ventricular Apical and Lateral Venous Stimulation

Biventricular pacing from these sites typically causes a negative deflection in lead I or a right bundle branch block pattern in lead V_1, with a negative deflection (S wave) in leads II, III, and aVF. Biventricular pacing from these two sites can be difficult to distinguish from posterolateral venous pacing alone. Typically, with posterolateral venous pacing alone, lead II is more negative (deeper S wave) than lead III. With right ventricular pacing alone, lead III has deeper S waves than lead II. Biventricular stimulation from these sites results in nearly equal negativity in leads II and III. This pattern in conjunction with a negative deflection in lead I, which cannot occur with right ventricular pacing alone, suggests biventricular stimulation and capture.

Right Ventricular Apical and Middle Cardiac Vein Pacing Sites

Because of the relative proximity of the right ventricular apex and the main course of the middle cardiac vein, biventricular stimulation between these two sites is very difficult to distinguish from stimulation and capture of one site alone.[23,24] The most important clue in this situation is the simultaneous presence of a right bundle branch block pattern in an otherwise difficult pattern of right ventricular apical pacing (i.e., a negative deflection in leads II, III, and aVF, and a positive deflection in leads aVR and aVL). The relative depth of the S waves in leads II and III can also be used as discussed in the section above on right ventricular apical and lateral venous stimulation sites.

Other Right Ventricular Sites Along With Left Ventricular Stimulation

The ECGs in this situation are difficult to analyze for biventricular capture without previous knowledge of the right ventricular site. This situation is a frequent cause of error in misdiagnosing which lead is failing to capture. For example, when a high right ventricular septal site along with a middle cardiac vein site for left ventricular stimulation is used when the left ventricular lead is failing to capture, then positive R waves in leads II, III, and aVF will be seen from the high septal right ventricular stimulation site.[5] The positive deflection in lead III and the other inferior leads will give the mistaken impression of left ventricular pacing and wrongly suggest failure to capture of the right ventricular lead. Present devices that allow separate stimulation of the left ventricular and right ventricular leads have greatly simplified diagnosing appropriate ventricular lead capture during threshold testing. During routine follow-up with only the ECG available, it is vital to have previous ECGs or documentation of the exact site where the leads were placed at implantation.

Assessing Ventricular Synchrony With the ECG

The initial premise of biventricular pacing was that simultaneous stimulation of the right and left ventricles would lead to mechanical synchronization of ventricular function. It is clear that simultaneous stimulation from disparate sites in the right and left ventricles will shorten the total duration of the QRS complex (ventricular depolarization) and predict a shortened synchronization.[25] However, there are several situations in which an electrical synchronization does not predict mechanical synchronization. There may be significant or even extreme capture latency from a pacing site, that is, a time delay from the delivery of the pacing stimulus to ventricular capture diminishes the contribution to ventricular depolarization from that pacing site.[26] In an extreme situation, there is no difference between single-site pacing and dual-site stimulation with one site having extreme capture latency. Capture latency as well as exit delay from a particular pacing site may be manifest only at more rapid pacing rates because of the decremental properties of the myocardium in certain diseases. Similarly, if stimulation is performed from a site, for example, in the left ventricle, that is close to scarred or diseased myocardium, the relative contribution to global ventricular depolarization from that pacing site will be minimal (Fig. 12).[27]

The contribution of one pacing site to overall ventricular capture can be estimated by comparing the 12-lead ECG with biventricular pacing with the ECG of pacing from the individual stimulation sites.[28] If the biventricular-paced ECG (with capture confirmed with individual lead testing) is similar to right ventricular pacing alone, it suggests that the left ventricular lead is not contributing to ventricular depolarization. This could be due to capture latency or extreme delay in exiting from the local myocardial capture at the site of the lead. If this situation is recognized at implantation, an attempt should be made to move the lead to a different site. If this is found at follow-up after implantation and the capability for varying the ventricle-to-ventricle stimulation timing is available, the timing should be set to pace earlier in the lead that is contributing less to ventricular depolarization.[29] For example, if the biventricular-paced ECG approximates the right ventricular pacing ECG, then left ventricular timing should be made to precede right ventricular timing.

The QRS duration has been used to determine whether ventricular synchronization is occurring (Fig. 3),[3] but using the QRS duration alone has pitfalls. Right ventricular septal pacing may produce a more narrow QRS complex than the

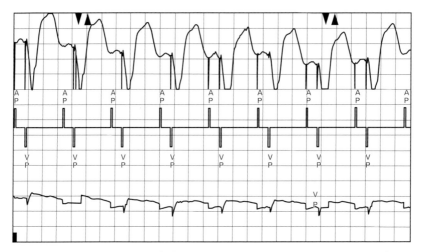

Figure 12. Subtle changes in the QRS morphology can sometimes be seen on careful analysis without change in the pacing output. This is usually seen at or near threshold. Reasons for this include anodal stimulation where there is a transient change in the vector of stimulation, and in severely diseased hearts, variable degrees of exit delay from the left ventricular pacing site (presumably within markedly diseased tissue) result in varying degrees of fusion.

addition of a left ventricular lead.[11] This may be due to functional refractoriness of the left ventricle caused by left ventricular stimulation producing an overall delay in total ventricular activation.

In addition to the above-mentioned caveat for using QRS duration as a surrogate for ventricular synchronization, the following need to be considered. Portions of the QRS may be isoelectric with biventricular pacing because of the summated vectors of different sites such as the right ventricular apex and an anterior interventricular vein site. This may give a false impression of a narrow QRS complex when in fact portions of the QRS complex are not identified on the 12-lead ECG.[23,24] This error is compounded when one or only a few leads are used to measure the QRS complex. Perhaps more importantly, it is well recognized that mechanical synchronization is not necessarily implied by electrical synchronization, because electrical activation at a particular site variably produces contraction depending on the electromechanical coupling interval.[30] This interval, in turn, depends on various factors, including ischemia, scar tissue, dysplasia, and fiber orientation. Despite these limitations, if the ECG is analyzed accurately, it can give an approximate idea of resynchronization (Fig. 13 and 14).

In summary, the 12-lead ECG should be analyzed first for a decrease in QRS duration with biventricular pacing. This suggests that global depolarization is being shortened with the use of the two sites. Next, the biventricular ECG should be compared with the ECG from pacing at individual sites. The dual-site stimulation ECG

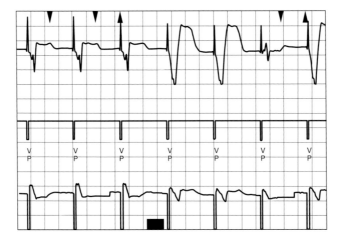

Figure 13. Biventricular, posterolateral vein to right ventricle only. Lead III QRS complexes are seen while pacing output is being decreased. The first three complexes show biventricular capture. The next two complexes show loss of capture from the left ventricular lead, giving rise to right ventricular stimulation only. The next complex is a fusion beat between right ventricular pacing and intrinsic conduction. Note widening of the QRS complex when biventricular capture is lost. Lead III continues to be negative with or without biventricular stimulation. This suggests that the left ventricular pacing lead is located in a posterior or posterolateral location, that is, the middle cardiac or posterolateral vein. However, the degree of QRS narrowing during biventricular stimulation suggests that the lead is in fact in the posterolateral vein, resulting in better synchronization and shortening of the QRS complex than is likely from the middle cardiac vein.

should be a vector of some of the individual pacing site ECGs. If the biventricular ECG is similar to either right or left ventricular pacing alone, it suggests that the lead that is not manifest with biventricular pacing is not contributing to global depolarization significantly. Either lead repositioning or ventricle-to-ventricle timing should be adjusted to produce better evidence of a balanced biventricular contribution to ventricular depolarization.

Biatrial Pacing

The ECG principles outlined above are equally applicable to atrial pacing. The P wave vector from right atrial appendage pacing results in a positive P wave in lead I, a negative wave in leads aVR and V_1, and a positive wave in leads II, III, and aVF. Pacing from the coronary sinus ostium, as with dual-site atrial pacing, typically results in a biphasic or negative P wave in leads II, III, and aVF and a biphasic initially positive and then negative deflection in lead V_1. Left atrial pacing, for example, from a lateral atrial vein such as the vein of Marshall, produces a negative P wave in leads I and aVL.

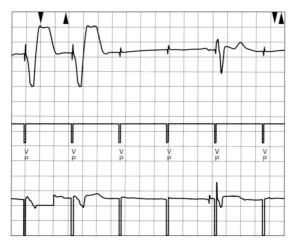

Figure 14. Further decrease in the output results in loss of right ventricular capture, and the intrinsic complex can be seen. Often, the intrinsic complexes seen soon after loss of capture are narrow compared with the native QRS complexes seen before pacing was initiated. This likely is due to retrograde penetration bilaterally of the bundle branch system giving rise to equal delay when intrinsic conduction comes through, relatively normalizing the QRS complex.

Coronary Sinus Musculature

The musculature of the coronary sinus is continuous with the right atrium. Very proximal locations for attempting ventricular pacing in a ventricular vein occasionally may stimulate the local atrial myocardial extension into the coronary sinus, resulting in atrial activation that in turn may activate the ventricle. This may be mistakenly interpreted as local ventricular capture. Although this situation is rare, ventricular activation may also occur because of coronary sinus musculature via a closely related but different ventricular vein than where the pacing lead is located. This will result in slight, usually subtle, changes in the ECG pattern during pacing from a particular location. This may be mistakenly interpreted as loss of capture. This misinterpretation can be avoided by paying careful attention to all details of the ECG.

Examples

Example 1 (Fig. 15 and 16)

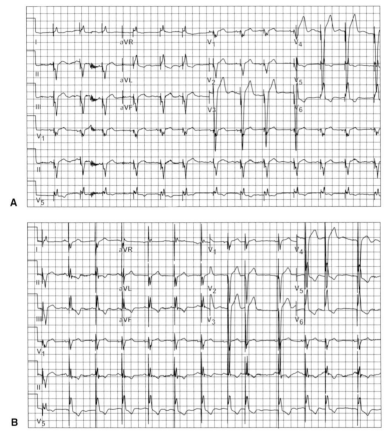

Figure 15. The classic pattern with right ventricular pacing from the right ventricular apex is shown in A. A left bundle branch block morphology with negative deflections in leads II, III, and aVF and a tall R wave in lead I and aVL all signify right ventricular apical pacing. Biventricular capture is seen in B (after the first beat). There is a dramatic shortening in the QRS complex and a marked change in the vector. Lead I now becomes negative, suggesting lateral ventricular stimulation, and leads II, III, and aVF become positive, suggesting an anterior location. Note that despite the anterolateral rather than straight lateral location, excellent shortening of the QRS duration is seen. The 9th, 11th, and 12th beats in B are premature atrial contractions with biventricular capture. Note that the QRS complex is slightly more prolonged with the faster pacing rate triggered by the premature atrial contractions in patients with ventricular conduction abnormalities or those taking antiarrhythmic drugs. This effect can be pronounced. This is one of the limitations to biventricular pacing in patients with atrial fibrillation and relatively rapid ventricular responses necessitating rapid pacing rates.

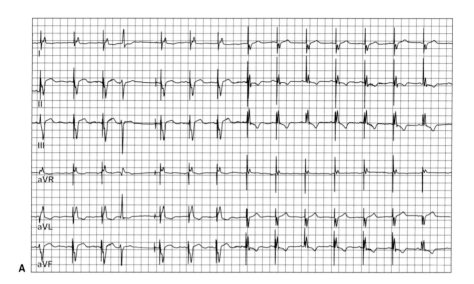

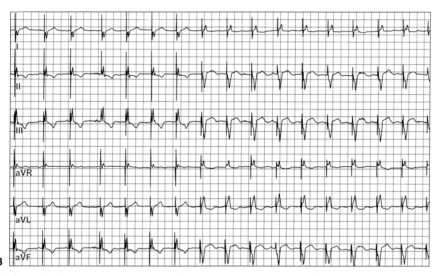

Figure 16. The same example as in Figure 15 showing the effect of increasing the pacing output (A) and then decreasing it (B). Because of the given lead position in this example, any one of the leads can be used to quickly see whether biventricular stimulation is occurring. For example, the negativity in lead I and the positivity in lead III are easily observed when increasing the output and obtaining left ventricular stimulation.

Example 2 (Fig. 17)

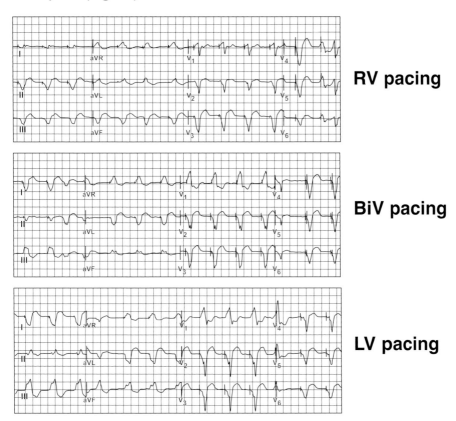

RV pacing

BiV pacing

LV pacing

Figure 17. This example illustrates the importance of systematic analysis of biventricular (BiV) tracings. With right ventricular (RV) pacing, a relatively characteristic morphology is seen, with a left bundle branch block pattern and negative deflections in leads II, III, and aVF. However, careful analysis shows an early small positive deflection in lead V_1 and varying degrees of QRS widening, especially evident in lead V_2. Both these findings suggest conduction abnormalities at the RV exit site. With left ventricular (LV) pacing, a characteristic right bundle branch block pattern with negative deflections in leads I and aVL is seen. The QRS vector is upright in the inferior leads (leads II, III, and aVF). This suggests that the LV pacing lead has been placed in a lateral vein in a slightly anterior location. BiV pacing results in an ECG that is very similar to LV pacing alone. This suggests that the RV lead is contributing little to the overall pacing vector. Thus, there is no added shortening of the QRS complex duration, a surrogate for resynchronization when adding RV pacing to LV pacing alone. In such instances, the availability of varying the ventricle-to-ventricle stimulation interval (VV timing) will allow better QRS shortening. In this instance, stimulating the RV earlier than the LV lead will approximate simultaneous stimulation of the ventricles. This ability to vary the VV timing may be more important when there is LV delay and the BiV-paced QRS morphology resembles RV pacing alone. This is because QT dynamic data show similar benefits with LV pacing and BiV stimulation.

Example 3 (Fig. 18)

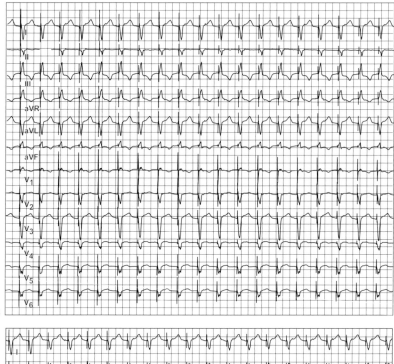

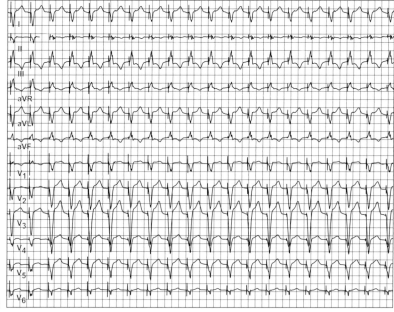

See legend on next page.

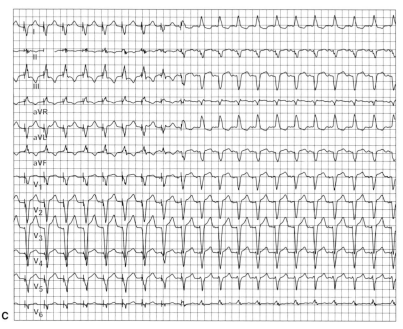

C

Figure 18. A-C, This series of ECGs illustrates the difficulty with using a single lead to assess left ventricular capture thresholds. Biventricular stimulation is seen in A. B shows that with decreasing the output of this biventricular system, a change in morphology occurs after the first two QRS complexes. The question is, which lead has lost capture? Is it the right ventricular or the left ventricular pacing lead? C shows that further decrease in the output voltage results in the loss of capture altogether, and intrinsic rhythm with left bundle branch block ensues. If one is asked to assess whether the right or left ventricular lead has lost capture (B), it would be nearly impossible to answer this question from analysis of lead III alone because lead III continues to be positive. This suggests that the right ventricular lead (usually resulting in negative complexes in lead III) has lost capture. However, in lead V_1, the resulting QRS complexes are negative (left bundle branch block pattern). In fact, the loss of capture was in the left ventricular lead. However, because the right ventricular lead had been placed in the high interventricular septum, the QRS complex is positive in lead III. Accurate knowledge of the position of the right ventricular lead and analysis of the entire 12-lead ECG are necessary with certain complicated circumstances.

References

1. Gras D, Leclercq C, Tang AS, Bucknall C, Luttikhuis HO, Kirstein-Pedersen A. Cardiac resynchronization therapy in advanced heart failure: the multicenter InSync clinical study. Eur J Heart Fail 2002;4:311-20.
2. Abraham WT. Cardiac resynchronization therapy for heart failure: biventricular pacing and beyond. Curr Opin Cardiol 2002;17:346-52.
3. Auricchio A, Stellbrink C, Sack S, Block M, Vogt J, Bakker P, et al. The Pacing Therapies for Congestive Heart Failure (PATH-CHF) study: rationale, design, and endpoints of a prospective randomized multicenter study. Am J Cardiol 1999;83:130D-5D.
4. Kay GN, Bourge RC. Biventricular pacing for congestive heart failure: questions of who, what, where, why, how, and how much. Am Heart J 2000;140:821-3.
5. Thompson C, Tsiperfal A. Why does the QRS morphology of the paced beat change in patients with biventricular cardiac pacing systems? Prog Cardiovasc Nurs 2002;17:101, 103.
6. Alonso C, Leclercq C, Victor F, Mansour H, de Place C, Pavin D, et al. Electrocardiographic predictive factors of long-term clinical improvement with multisite biventricular pacing in advanced heart failure. Am J Cardiol 1999;84:1417-21.
7. Daoud EG, Kalbfleisch SJ, Hummel JD, Weiss R, Augustini RS, Duff SB, et al. Implantation techniques and chronic lead parameters of biventricular pacing dual-chamber defibrillators. J Cardiovasc Electrophysiol 2002;13:964-70.
8. Willems JL, Lesaffre E. Comparison of multigroup logistic and linear discriminant ECG and VCG classification. J Electrocardiol 1987;20:83-92.
9. Willems JL, Lesaffre E, Pardaens J. Comparison of the classification ability of the electrocardiogram and vectorcardiogram. Am J Cardiol 1987;59:119-24.
10. Bortolan G, Willems JL. Diagnostic ECG classification based on neural networks. J Electrocardiol 1993;26 Suppl:75-9.
11. Brohet CR, Robert A, Derwael C, Fesler R, Stijns M, Vliers A, et al. Computer interpretation of pediatric orthogonal electrocardiograms: statistical and deterministic classification methods. Circulation 1984;70:255-62.
12. Kornreich F, Block P, Brismee D. The missing waveform information in the orthogonal electrocardiogram (Frank leads): IV. computer diagnosis of biventricular hypertrophy from "maximal" surface waveform information. Circulation 1974;49:1123-31.
13. Kulbertus HE, de Laval-Rutten F, Casters P. Vectorcardiographic study of aberrant conduction anterior displacement of QRS: another form of intraventricular block. Br Heart J 1976;38:549-57.
14. Wyman BT, Hunter WC, Prinzen FW, Faris OP, McVeigh ER. Effects of single- and biventricular pacing on temporal and spatial dynamics of ventricular contraction. Am J Physiol Heart Circ Physiol 2002;282:H372-9.
15. Farrar DJ, Chow E, Wood JR, Hill JD. Anatomic interaction between the right and left ventricles during univentricular and biventricular circulatory support. ASAIO Trans 1988;34:235-40.
16. Jain A, Chandna H, Silber EN, Clark WA, Denes P. Electrocardiographic patterns of patients with echocardiographically determined biventricular hypertrophy. J Electrocardiol 1999;32:269-73.
17. Igarashi M, Shiina Y, Tanabe T, Handa S. Significance of electrocardiographic QRS width in patients with congestive heart failure: a marker for biventricular pacing [Japanese]. J Cardiol 2002;40:103-9.

18. Cazeau S, Ritter P, Lazarus A, Gras D, Backdach H, Mundler O, et al. Multisite pacing for end-stage heart failure: early experience. Pacing Clin Electrophysiol 1996;19:1748-57.

19. Lehmann A, Lang J, Thaler E, Zeitler C, Weisse U, Boldt J. Considerations in patients undergoing implantation of a biventricular pacemaker. J Cardiothorac Vasc Anesth 2002;16:175-9.

20. Touiza A, Etienne Y, Gilard M, Fatemi M, Mansourati J, Blanc JJ. Long-term left ventricular pacing: assessment and comparison with biventricular pacing in patients with severe congestive heart failure. J Am Coll Cardiol 2001;38:1966-70.

21. Yong P, Duby C. A new and reliable method of individual ventricular capture identification during biventricular pacing threshold testing. Pacing Clin Electrophysiol 2000;23:1735-7.

22. Manyari DE, Kostuk WJ, Klein GJ, Guiraudon G, Purves P. Local right ventricular electrogram for ECG-gated cardioscintigraphy to assess right ventricular function during biventricular dissociation. Am Heart J 1984;107:385-8.

23. Reuter S, Garrigue S, Bordachar P, Hocini M, Jais P, Haissaguerre M, et al. Intermediate-term results of biventricular pacing in heart failure: correlation between clinical and hemodynamic data. Pacing Clin Electrophysiol 2000;23:1713-7.

24. Ricci R, Pignalberi C, Ansalone G, Jannone E, Vaccaro MV, Denaro A, et al. Early and late QRS morphology and width in biventricular pacing: relationship to lead site and electrical remodeling. J Interv Card Electrophysiol 2002;6:279-85.

25. Ansalone G, Giannantoni P, Ricci R, Trambaiolo P, Fedele F, Santini M. Doppler myocardial imaging to evaluate the effectiveness of pacing sites in patients receiving biventricular pacing. J Am Coll Cardiol 2002;39:489-99.

26. O'Cochlain B, Delurgio D, Leon A, Langberg J. The effect of variation in the interval between right and left ventricular activation on paced QRS duration. Pacing Clin Electrophysiol 2001;24:1780-2.

27. Contini C, Berti S, Levorato D, Bongiorni MG, Baratto MT, Arlotta C, et al. Histologic evidence of myocardial damage in apparently healthy subjects with ventricular arrhythmias and myocardial dysfunction. Clin Cardiol 1992;15:529-33.

28. Pitzalis MV, Iacoviello M, Romito R, Massari F, Rizzon B, Luzzi G, et al. Cardiac resynchronization therapy tailored by echocardiographic evaluation of ventricular asynchrony. J Am Coll Cardiol 2002;40:1615-22.

29. Prinzen FW, Van Oosterhout MF, Vanagt WY, Storm C, Reneman RS. Optimization of ventricular function by improving the activation sequence during ventricular pacing. Pacing Clin Electrophysiol 1998;21:2256-60.

30. Breithardt OA, Stellbrink C, Kramer AP, Sinha AM, Franke A, Salo R, et al., PATH-CHF Study Group. Echocardiographic quantification of left ventricular asynchrony predicts an acute hemodynamic benefit of cardiac resynchronization therapy. J Am Coll Cardiol 2002;40:536-45.

CHAPTER 4

Biventricular Device Implantation

Samuel J. Asirvatham, MD

Introduction

Familiarity with placing left ventricular leads as part of biventricular device implantation is becoming increasingly necessary.[1,2] This chapter focuses on the technical details of cannulating the coronary sinus and effectively deploying a left ventricular lead. It is assumed that the reader is facile with standard pacemaker and implantable cardioverter-defibrillator lead placement.[3] Issues germane to usual lead placement are discussed only if they directly affect the successful placement of a left ventricular lead. First, the general considerations for the technique involved are outlined. Second, commonly encountered difficulties are discussed and solutions suggested. Third, an algorithm is presented, with suggestions for a stepwise approach for difficult cases. It is also imperative that the implanting physician have a thorough knowledge of coronary venous anatomy (Fig. 1-3).

General Considerations

A working knowledge of device implantation is assumed. However, certain features of the routine implant may require specific consideration when placing a left ventricular lead.

Side of Implant

Left ventricular leads may be deployed by either a right- or left-sided implant. In this chapter, the description for lead manipulation and sheath selection is for a left-sided implant. It is incorrect to assume that opposite maneuvers are required for a right-sided implant. In fact, because of the additional curve between the axis of the subclavian vein and the superior vena cava on the right side, identical results are obtained with similar maneuvers. For example, counterclockwise torque applied to

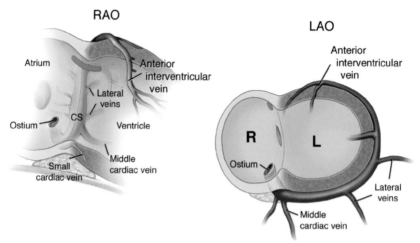

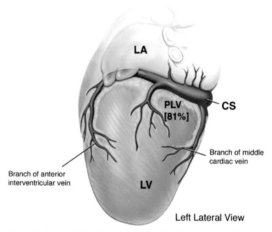

Figure 1. Coronary sinus (CS) and ventricular vein anatomy ideally are visualized in two orthogonal fluoroscopic views. In the right anterior oblique (RAO) projection, the CS is viewed end-on. The ostium of the CS is just superior to the usually visualized translucency of the posterior fat pad. The body of the CS and great cardiac vein proceed end-on, separating the ventricles and atria. In this projection, the ventricular veins then proceed toward the sternum. In the left anterior oblique (LAO) projection, the ostium of CS is in the plane of the interatrial septum. The vein proceeds posteriorly from right to left, wrapping around the lateral wall of the heart. In this view, atrial and ventricular veins cannot be distinguished, which they easily can be in the RAO projection. The LAO projection is ideal for distinguishing lateral and septal locations of veins and contained leads.

Figure 2. The lateral left ventricle (LV) is drained by branches of the posterolateral vein (PLV) in most patients. It should be noted that lateral branches of the anterior intraventricular vein and lateral branches of the middle cardiac vein also drain this region. CS, coronary sinus; LA, left atrium.

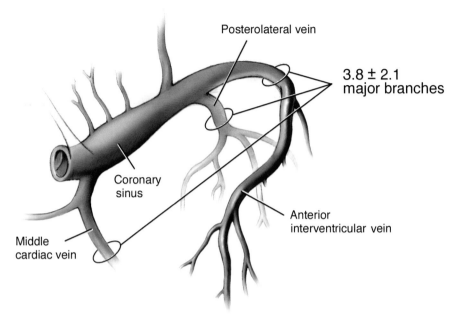

Posterolateral vein

3.8 ± 2.1
major branches

Coronary
sinus

Anterior
interventricular vein

Middle
cardiac vein

Figure 3. Ventricular venous anatomy. Three to four ventricular veins are seen fairly consistently. The middle cardiac vein can be either close to or widely separated from the posterolateral vein. When the posterolateral vein is close to the middle cardiac vein, lateral branches of the anterior intraventricular vein or a separate lateral vein drain the left ventricular free wall.

a sheath or lead will deflect the tip of the lead or sheath toward the septum and in an atrial direction. Clockwise torque causes a more ventricular and free-wall orientation of the tip. This is true both for right- and left-sided implants. Specific differences in manipulation for the right side are pointed out below.

Venous Access

A coronary sinus lead can be placed with venous access through subclavian venipuncture, cephalic vein cutdown, extrathoracic subclavian venipuncture, or axillary venipuncture. For placing a left ventricular lead, it is often vital to be able to impart graded and sometimes extensive torque to cannulate the coronary sinus and to subselect coronary veins.[4] Thus, medial subclavian punctures should be avoided as lead maneuverability can be difficult. The author prefers to perform either extrathoracic subclavian or axillary vein puncture to maximize sheath and lead mobility. Also, it has been recommended that multiple lead placement through a single venipuncture site be avoided because of the propensity for lead dislodgement while manipulating the non–left ventricular leads; an increase in backbleeding and difficulty with sheath or left ventricular lead manipulation (or both) may be noted.

Sequence of Placing Leads

The left ventricular lead may be placed before or after the right ventricular and right atrial leads have been placed. The advantages of placing the left ventricular lead first include the greater ease in maneuvering the guiding sheath and lead, partial occlusion of the orifice of the coronary sinus with the ventricular lead, and inadvertent manipulation in the coronary sinus with the right ventricular lead, resulting in either spasm or dissection. Furthermore, if the implant is performed solely for biventricular pacing, the inability to place the left ventricular lead causes unnecessary deployment of the other leads. The major advantages of placing the right ventricular lead first include a fixed reference to the apex and tricuspid annulus and ventricular pacing support if the patient has extensive conduction system disease.

As explained below, the right anterior oblique (RAO) projection is used to define the tricuspid valve annulus, and the left anterior oblique (LAO) projection is used to define the interventricular septum and apex. In patients with dilated cardiac chambers, the "usual" amount of RAO and LAO to achieve this orientation may differ greatly. The characteristic change in the contour of the right ventricular lead at the tricuspid annulus and its placement at the apex can help to line up these views in a patient.

If a temporary transvenous pacing catheter is placed from the femoral vein, clockwise torque to obtain a septal placement of this lead may also help define the ideal LAO angle. The author prefers to place the left ventricular lead first. In difficult cases, particularly with asymmetric dilatation of the left ventricle or clockwise rotation of the heart (or both), the right ventricular lead should be placed at the apex first to provide optimal orientation.

Previous Implantation

Frequently, preexisting pacemakers and defibrillators require an upgrade to a biventricular system, which requires placing a left ventricular lead. Fibrosis and partial occlusions of the subclavian brachiocephalic-superior vena cava access can make left ventricular lead placement challenging. If the proximal portion of the axillary or subclavian vein is cannulated but standard guide wires or the sheath do not advance to the right atrium, the following steps should be considered: 1) direct contrast venography performed from the subclavian insertion site, 2) a deformable soft-tip wire such as the angled Glide wire can often negotiate partial occlusions successfully and advance to the inferior vena cava, 3) a long 6F sheath can be advanced over the Glide wire, 4) the Glide wire can be exchanged for a more supportive soft-tip but stiff-bodied wire such as the extra stiff Amplatz or Supracore wire, and 5) with such a wire placed in the inferior vena cava, the guiding sheath can be safely advanced, while pulling back on the wire as the sheath is advanced to the right atrium. If maneuverability of the sheath is limited after placement, both lead placement and removal of the sheath can be tenuous. The stiff-bodied wire can then be replaced through the sheath, the sheath can be serially dilated so it is two French sizes larger, and the guiding sheath reintroduced. A loosely tied purse-string suture may be required around the insertion site to control perisheath bleeding.

Coronary Sinus Cannulation

Once venous access has been established, the coronary sinus must be cannulated with a guiding sheath. The ventricular lead is deployed through the sheath, after which the sheath is removed. This stage is critical for successful implantation of a biventricular device. Attention to detail and experience in troubleshooting problems that arise with cannulating the coronary sinus will decrease procedure time and minimize coronary sinus-related complications.[5]

The Guiding Sheath

Several varieties of guiding sheaths are available but there are major differences in shape and method of sheath removal. Straight sheaths with no preformed curves typically require a deflectable catheter for initial cannulation of the coronary sinus. Preformed curves are available in several varieties; no one curve is ideally suited for all hearts. Generally, gentle curves are preferred to give flexibility if subselection of a coronary vein is required or multiple catheter exchanges are needed to cannulate the coronary sinus. If a preformed curved sheath is used, the coronary sinus can be engaged with either an angiographic wire or a deflectable catheter. When a large right atrium is encountered, an Amplatz-like curve in the sheath or the creation of a similar curve in the sheath with a deflectable catheter can be beneficial. Cannulation of the middle cardiac vein should not be attempted with sheaths that have sharp primary or secondary curves (see below).

Use of Angiographic Wires Versus Deflectable Electrophysiologic Catheters to Engage the Coronary Sinus

Angiographic wires that are soft-tipped and torquable are well suited for use with preshaped guiding sheaths.[6-8] To engage the coronary sinus, the wire is advanced preferably as far as the natural curve of the coronary sinus, great cardiac vein, anterior vein, and interventricular vein will allow. The guiding sheath is then advanced along the wire while the wire is pulled back. The sheath should not be advanced when the wire has not freely advanced into the axis of the coronary veins. This is to avoid coronary sinus dissection. If the wire has not advanced sufficiently to allow it to be pulled back a substantial amount while the sheath is being advanced, then repeatedly pulling back the wire and readvancing the sheath in small increments will allow the coronary sinus to be safely engaged with the guiding sheath (Fig. 4).

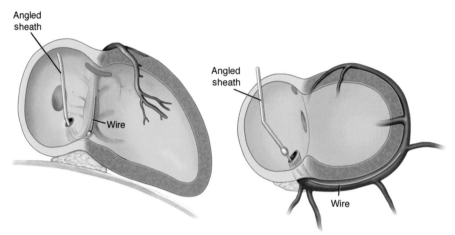

Figure 4. Cannulating the coronary sinus with a guide wire. The use of a curved or angled sheath guide wire can be used to engage the coronary sinus and its tributaries. With the sheath rotated counterclockwise so that it points septally in the left anterior oblique projection, the wire is advanced gently, and it is seen to take the typical course of the vein in both the right and left anterior oblique projections.

Deflectable electrophysiologic catheters can be used with either straight or preformed curved guiding sheaths. The author prefers to use deflectable catheters capable of recording electrograms and whose deflection mechanism allows bidirectional changes. After the coronary sinus has been cannulated, pulling back on the catheter slightly while advancing the sheath will allow the sheath to be deployed into the coronary sinus (Fig. 5-7).

In most cases, either technique—angiographic wires or deflectable electrophysiologic catheters—is successful. The advantage of angiographic wires is that their small size and soft tip allow repeated advancements into the appropriate radiographic planes; also, they engage and advance through tortuous, small-diameter, or partially dissected coronary veins. If the eustachian ridge is prominent, the guiding sheath needs to be placed ventricularly to the ridge to allow the wire to engage the coronary sinus. This can be a difficult maneuver. Deflectable electrophysiologic catheters have the advantage of recording electrograms, which should show a balanced atrial and ventricular signal to identify annular locations in the patient. Furthermore, catheters with bidirectional curves can be used to negotiate sharp bends over prominent eustachian ridges and around near circumferential thebesian valves.[9] In choosing between these two techniques, the operator should make the decision on the basis of his or her experience (Fig. 8). For example, an interventionalist may prefer trying various wires, whereas an electrophysiologist is likely to be more comfortable with deflectable catheters. Regardless, deflectable catheters

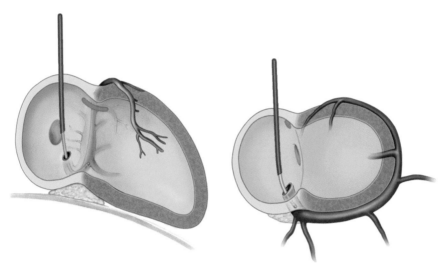

Figure 5. Either straight or curved sheaths can be used with a deflectable catheter to engage the coronary sinus. The catheter is deflected just above the posterior fat pad in an end-on manner in the right anterior oblique projection and points septally and leftward in the left anterior oblique projection. Care should be taken that once the catheter has engaged the coronary sinus, the sheath should be advanced to the ostium of the coronary sinus with gentle pulling back of the catheter (see text).

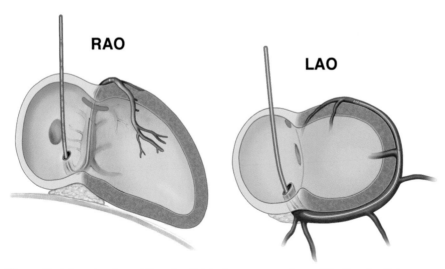

Figure 6. Advancing the guiding sheath into the coronary sinus. After the sheath has been placed in the ostium of the coronary sinus, the deflectable catheter is advanced to the region of the desired vein. While pulling back on the catheter, advance the sheath and then advance the catheter again. Repeat this maneuver until the desired location in the venous system has been obtained. LAO, left anterior oblique; RAO, right anterior oblique.

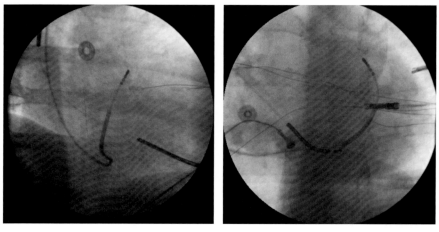

Figure 7. Left, Right anterior oblique and, right, left anterior oblique projections showing cannulation of the great cardiac vein using a deflectable catheter.

are larger in diameter and may not allow cannulation in patients with coronary vein stenosis, spasm, or extremely tortuous veins. It is imperative that minimal force be applied with slow and gentle movements because coronary sinus dissection is more likely with larger catheters, especially if care is not taken with the manipulation. This risk is minimized if the operator avoids advancing the sheath when the tip of

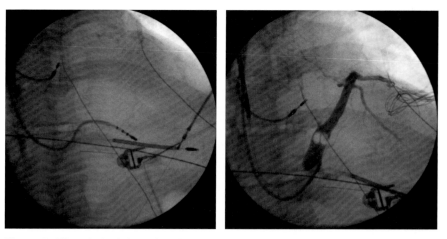

Figure 8. When desired, the deflectable catheter can be used to subselect the vein of interest and, using the maneuver described above, the sheath can be advanced into the ventricular vein. Note that angiography failed to visualize the branch that was located with gentle probing with the deflectable catheter.

the catheter is not free, avoids advancing into atrial coronary veins, and matches the French size of the catheter with the sheath.

Ostial Placement of the Guiding Sheath Versus Subselection Into a Ventricular Vein

With either an angiographic wire or an electrophysiologic deflectable catheter, the sheath can be advanced into the main body of the coronary sinus or subselectively into a ventricular vein. With the availability of over-the-wire left ventricular leads, ostial placement of the sheath is usually sufficient. Occasionally, it can be difficult to maneuver a lead into a desired branch, especially if an over-the-wire system is not used (see below). This is particularly true when trying to engage the middle cardiac vein.[10] In these instances, a deflectable catheter can be used to subselect the vein of interest. With the use of the RAO projection, the catheter is deflected to point in the ventricular direction. From the most distal location to which the catheter can be advanced with this ventricular orientation, the catheter is pulled back slowly while the torque is changed over approximately 15 degrees, alternating in a clockwise and counterclockwise direction. With this maneuver, the ostium of a ventricular vein (anterolateral, lateral, or posterolateral vein) will be engaged. After the ostium has been engaged, the sheath should be advanced to approximately 1 cm proximal to the orifice of the vein. Next, the deflectable catheter is gently advanced into the vein as distally as possible. While care is taken to pull back on the catheter, the sheath is advanced subselectively into the ventricular vein. The ventricular lead then can usually be advanced into the vein without difficulty.

To subselect the middle cardiac vein, the following technique may be used. Initially, the catheter and sheath need to be rotated counterclockwise to enter the coronary sinus. After the coronary sinus has been entered with the deflectable catheter, the sheath is removed just atrial to the ostium of the coronary sinus. The deflectable catheter is then curved, and clockwise torque is applied to point the tip of the catheter in a ventricular direction using the RAO imaging plane. The catheter is drawn back gently, while clockwise rotation continues to be applied, when a characteristic jump to a ventricular position will be seen. It may be difficult to discern whether the catheter has advanced into the middle cardiac vein or the right ventricle. In the LAO projection, deflection should be performed in at least two planes to show that the catheter does not move freely, suggesting placement into a venous structure. The sheath, which is now in the right atrium, should be aligned as much as possible at a straight angle to the catheter in the middle cardiac vein and gently advanced while the catheter is drawn into the body of the middle cardiac vein. It is critical that this maneuver not be used while the guiding sheath is still in the main body of the coronary sinus because the sharp angle that is needed to engage this vein is likely to cause proximal dissections in the middle cardiac vein and ostium of the coronary sinus, precluding further efforts to place a left ventricular lead.

Coronary Sinus Angiography

After the guiding sheath has been placed at the ostium of the coronary sinus, coronary venography may be performed (Fig. 9).[6-8] Coronary sinus angiography can be performed effectively with end-hole balloon-tipped catheters (with injection of the contrast dye through the guiding sheath with or without a balloon on the sheath) or with deflectable electrophysiologic catheters that allow the injection of contrast dye (Daig multielectrode lumen, Irvine Biomedical Systems). The technique most commonly used is balloon occlusion angiography. Care should be taken that the tip of the balloon catheter is free; the catheter should be advanced approximately 1 cm beyond the guiding sheath. If further advancement is not possible, the catheter should be pulled back to a point where the tip is clearly free before the injection of contrast dye is contemplated. The balloon is then inflated and gently pulled back to the guiding sheath. Complete deployment of the balloon aids visualization of the

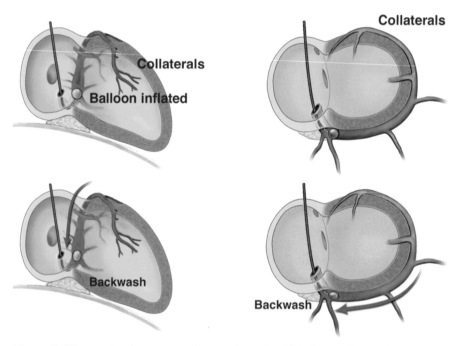

Figure 9. When performing coronary sinus angiography with balloon catheters, the distal coronary sinus, great cardiac vein, and ventricular veins are best visualized with complete inflation of the balloon and occlusion of the coronary sinus. More proximal branches and the middle cardiac vein can be visualized when collaterals reforming these veins are seen or with continuous imaging when the balloon is deflated and the ostia of the proximal veins are visualized with a backwash of contrast.

distal coronary venous tree (Fig. 10). The contrast agent is injected under cine flu-oroscopy. The anatomy of the coronary venous tree is visualized in at least two orthogonal planes, usually the RAO and LAO projections.[11,12] To obtain maximal anatomical information from balloon angiography, it is important that 1) complete occlusion is performed, 2) injection and cine fluoroscopy are continued until more proximal veins are seen to fill through anastomoses, and 3) fluoroscopy is contin-ued after the balloon has been deflated, because the backwash of contrast dye often demonstrates the ostia of the middle cardiac vein, proximal posterolateral veins, and the small cardiac vein.

Performed in this way, contrast coronary sinus venography provides a map for fur-ther manipulations of the ventricular lead (Fig. 11 and 12). However, coronary sinus angiography is not without limitations. First, if care is not taken to free the tip of the catheter before the injection of contrast dye, coronary sinus dissection or perforation (or both) will result. Second, in some patients, the contrast dye may adversely affect renal function or cause pulmonary edema. Third, the sheath may become dislodged during manipulation of the balloon catheter. Although coronary sinus angiography is helpful in some cases, effective lead deployment, especially with over-the-wire leads, can be accomplished without coronary sinus angiography. It probably is beneficial for an operator to use coronary sinus angiography for the first 20 to 30 implants to become familiar with coronary venous anatomy and to correlate this anatomy with fluoroscop-ic views and the "feel" of the lead engaging a particular vein. The author prefers to place the ventricular lead without performing coronary sinus angiography.

If it is difficult to select a vein and obtain adequate thresholds, angiography is performed and additional venous ostia are sought. If angiography is performed, the initial ventricular venous branch that is visualized with the injection of contrast dye

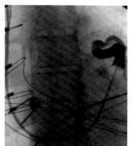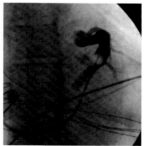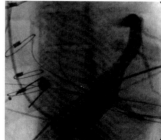

Figure 10. At times during coronary sinus angiography, visualization is best with a graded pullback technique. Initially, the balloon is placed distally and the distal vessels visualized. The balloon is then deflated more proximally to visualize mid-level branches. Either during the backwash phase or with gradual deflation of the balloon while pulling back the catheter, proximal ventricular as well as atrial branches can be visualized. This technique can be useful with large coronary veins.

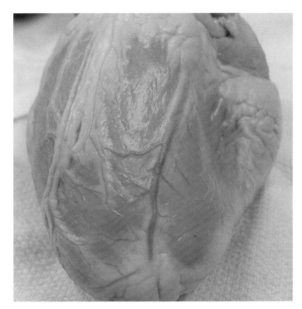

Figure 11. Autopsy specimen showing extensive anastomoses between the primary ventricular veins.

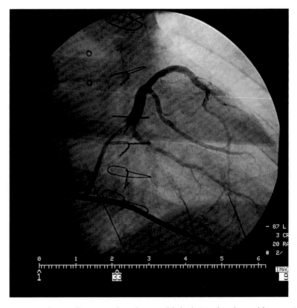

Figure 12. Coronary vein angiogram showing multiple lateral veins with anastomotic veins connecting the mid-lateral and anteriolateral veins.

often provides a clue to the direction the sheath is pointing. Repeated small injections while varying the torque on the sheath can align the sheath with a particular vein without necessarily subselecting that vein. If the question of possible dissection or perforation has already arisen, avoid performing angiography especially if the balloon catheter cannot be advanced freely to the main body of the coronary sinus or great cardiac vein. This may result in worsening of the dissection or perforation. It is imperative to avoid forceful injections because they may lead to dissection, perforation, or myocardial staining that may give rise to a malignant ventricular arrhythmia. Under no circumstance should power injectors be used for coronary sinus angiography.

Technique for Cannulating the Coronary Sinus

The primary imaging modality used for cannulation of the coronary sinus is fluoroscopy. Any projection is potentially useful to effectively engage the ostium of the coronary sinus. However, because of the angled location of the heart in the chest cavity, the true orthogonal views along the cardiac axes are the RAO and LAO projections (Fig. 13). The plane of viewing of the LAO projection is along the interventricular and interatrial septa. Therefore, the left side of the heart is viewed to our right and vice versa. In this projection, ventricular and atrial structures cannot be distinguished, but leftward and rightward and, thus, septal and free-wall locations can be distinguished clearly. In most hearts, an LAO projection angle of approximately 30 degrees will align along the interventricular septum. However, implantation of a biventricular device is often required for patients with grossly abnormal hearts. Therefore, certain deviations from this standard are required.[13] To define the septum in an asymmetrically enlarged heart, a catheter can be placed at the location where the His electrogram is recorded or the right ventricular pacing lead can be placed in the right ventricular apex. After the septum has been defined by one of these techniques, the LAO angle can be adjusted so that this septal catheter (His bundle or right ventricular apex) is viewed end-on. In particularly difficult cases, echocardiography can be used to define the location of the interventricular septum. It is not unusual that an LAO angle greater than 80 degrees is required to achieve the usual septal viewing plane. The natural viewing angle of the RAO projection is through the plane of the atrioventricular septum. With this viewing plane, it is easy to differentiate ventricular (i.e., toward the sternum) from atrial (i.e., toward the vertebral column) locations. Either of these viewing planes can easily distinguish superior and inferior locations.[14]

To locate the coronary sinus fluoroscopically, the following steps are performed: 1) In the RAO projection (approximately 30 degrees), the epicardial posteroseptal fat pad is visualized. This usually is seen near the angle of the right hemidiaphragm and the cardiac silhouette. If necessary, higher intensity fluoroscopy or higher frame rates can be used briefly to visualize the structure. Often, the annulus can be visualized as a relatively radiolucent area. Occasionally, stents

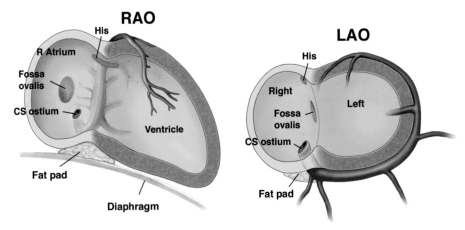

Figure 13. Important fluoroscopic and electrical landmarks include the fat pad of the pos-teroseptal space and the bundle of His. In the right anterior oblique (RAO) projection, the consistent landmark is the translucency between the hemidiaphragm and the cardiac silhou-ette caused by the fat pad of the posteroseptal space. Either the guidewire or a deflectable catheter can be aimed at this translucency. The wire or catheter is then advanced leftward from this space in the left anterior oblique (LAO) projection and in an end-on (appearing to come toward the operator) fashion in the RAO projection. In grossly distorted hearts, particu-larly with a large right (R) atrium, and in congenital anomalies, placing an electrical mapping catheter to locate the His bundle electrogram can help to define the interatrial septum. The catheter can be advanced toward the spine from this electrocardiogram with counterclock-wise torque to engage the coronary sinus (CS) ostium.

and coronary arterial calcifications define the annulus, as does a mechanoprosthetic cardiac atrioventricular valve. 2) The angiographic wire or deflectable electrophys-iologic catheter is moved to a location just posterior and cephalad to the epicardial posteroseptal fat pad. 3) Mild counterclockwise torque is applied to the catheter or sheath with wire, and the wire or catheter is gently advanced. 4) Now, the LAO viewing angle is used to ensure that the catheter or wire is advancing to the left side. 5) After the catheter or wire has advanced for approximately 1 to 2 cm into the coro-nary sinus (i.e., leftward in the LAO projection) and along the atrioventricular groove in the RAO projection, the sheath is advanced gently to engage the coronary sinus, as described above. Electrophysiologists who have placed several thousand coronary sinus catheters in patients with relatively normal hearts may be disoriented in the LAO projection in patients with grossly dilated left ventricles. As the left ven-tricle dilates, the angle of the coronary sinus becomes relatively more acute in the LAO projection. If subselection of a ventricular vein is contemplated (or atrial vein for left atrial pacing), the RAO projection is used to determine if the catheter or wire is advancing in a more ventricular or atrial direction.

Causes of Difficulty in Engaging the Coronary Sinus and Suggested Solutions

The Coronary Sinus Ostium and Course of the Coronary Sinus Are Not in the Expected Fluoroscopic Planes

This is the most common cause of difficulty because the wire or catheter does not advance in the usual location and angle as described above (Fig. 14).[15] Identifying the site of the His bundle with a characteristic His bundle electrogram or placing a catheter on the septum of the left ventricle to identify the degree of rotation or shift of the cardiac silhouette, with or without ultrasonography, is sometimes helpful. End-hole deflectable catheters, particularly those with electrodes, can be especially useful in this situation. When it appears or feels as if a venous structure has been entered with the catheter, gentle brief injections of contrast dye can be used to identify or exclude a venous channel. In particularly difficult cases, it is useful to visualize the coronary sinus with an alternate technique.[16] Arteriography of a left coronary artery—the left main, saphenous vein graft to a left-sided coronary artery or a left internal mammary graft—can be injected and the venous phase observed (Fig. 15). The venous phase typically lasts 10 to 15 seconds. With a single arterial injection during the venous phase, the fluoroscopic camera can be changed from an RAO to an LAO projection while a deflectable catheter is manipulated to engage the coronary sinus. Rarely are multiple injections required.

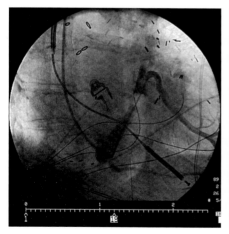 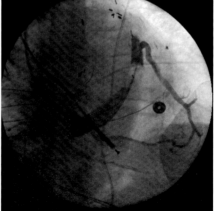

Figure 14. Left, Right anterior oblique and, right, left anterior obllique projections showing the typical takeoff of a lateral or posterolateral vein. Note the anastomosis between middle cardiac, posterior, and lateral veins.

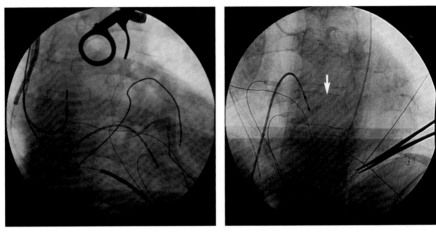

Figure 15. In this patient with grossly distorted cardiac anatomy in whom a previous attempt to engage the coronary sinus failed, coronary arteriography showed a nearly vertical coronary sinus (arrow) associated with surgically induced narrowing in the mid portion during the venous phase. Once visualized, appropriate maneuvers (see text) can be used to successfully negotiate the unusual takeoff and narrowing to obtain good lead position.

It is important to appreciate that right coronary angiography is not helpful in identifying the coronary sinus because right ventricular venous return may be exclusively through the thebesian vessels. Intracardiac ultrasonography with a 9F linear phased array catheter placed through the femoral vein into the right atrium can be used to identify the ostium of the coronary sinus as well as the course of the sinus.[17] After the catheter has been placed in the right atrium, the fluoroscopically darkened viewing transducer is visualized fluoroscopically and the catheter is rotated counterclockwise to view the tricuspid valve. Gentle clockwise rotation will bring the ostium of the coronary sinus into view.[18] If instead the fossa ovalis is seen, the catheter should be lowered with the same amount of torque to visualize the ostium of the coronary sinus. It is not always possible to obtain a view that shows the ostium and entire length of the coronary sinus, especially if there is a large eustachian ridge. If a large eustachian ridge precludes viewing the ostium of the coronary sinus, placing this catheter through the internal jugular vein may be considered. The catheter or wire being used to engage the coronary sinus is placed between the visualized transducer and the septum and advanced toward the left in the LAO projection.

Presence of a Large Right Atrium

In this situation, two approaches can be taken. One approach is to make a large curve with a deflectable electrophysiologic catheter to mimic an Amplatz-type curve or to use an Amplatz-shaped guiding sheath along with an angiographic wire. If an Amplatz-type sheath is used, the sheath should be placed relatively ventricularly to the fat pad in the RAO projection. Alternatively, the Amplatz-curved sheath can be directed to a ventricular orientation, and with gradual counterclockwise rotation and repeated advancement of a guide wire, the coronary sinus can be entered. The other approach is to use a straight sheath and a deflectable electrophysiologic catheter. With this technique, the sheath is advanced as septally as possible in the LAO orientation. The deflection mechanism of the catheter is deployed to engage the region of the fossa ovalis on the interatrial septum. After the catheter has been engaged, as will be evident with a leftward orientation in the LAO projection, it is advanced inferiorly. Thus, a typical bend is created, and by varying the deflection mechanism in a bidirectionally deflectable catheter and using gentle inferoposterior movements, the ostium of the coronary sinus can be located.[19] This maneuver is best performed in the LAO projection.

Thebesian Valve Prominence
A thebesian valve is found to various extents in patients.[20,21] It covers at least 50% of the orifice of the coronary sinus in approximately 20% of patients (Fig. 16-18). A prominent thebesian valve can make engagement of the coronary sinus challeng-

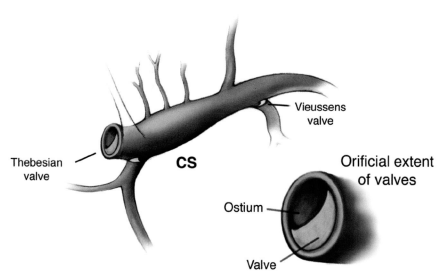

Figure 16. Venous valves can be found at various locations in the coronary sinus vasculature. The thebesian valve is the most consistent of these valves found at the orifice of the coronary sinus. The middle cardiac vein and posterolateral vein also may frequently be guarded by valves.

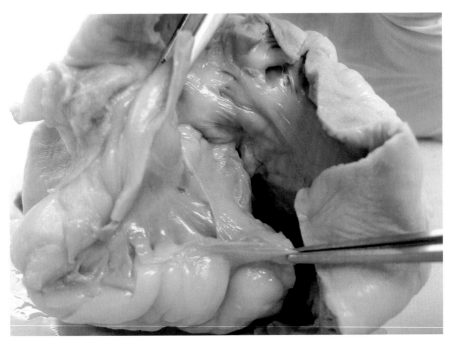

Figure 17. Autopsy specimen showing a large thebesian valve at the orifice of the coronary sinus. Note the numerous ventricular venous orifices close to the origin of the coronary sinus.

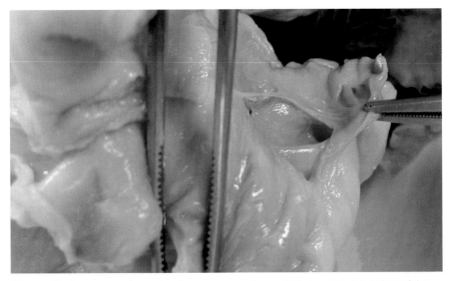

Figure 18. Autopsy specimen showing a venous valve partially covering the ostium of the middle cardiac vein.

ing. When this valve is prominent, it may cover primarily the superior or inferior portion of the coronary sinus. If the superior portion is covered, a straight or slightly curved sheath with a bidirectionally deflectable catheter can be used. When the usual fluoroscopic location of the coronary sinus is reached with the catheter, a backbend is deployed so as to bend the catheter with the tip facing the inferoposterior region of the atrium. If it appears that the ostium of the coronary sinus is hitched, the bend is released, thus virtually lifting up the thebesian valve, and the catheter and sheath are advanced in the usual fashion. If the thebesian valve primarily covers the inferior portion of the coronary sinus, a technique similar to that described with the straight sheath and engagement of the fossa ovalis, prolapsing the catheter into the coronary sinus, can be implemented.

If the thebesian valve is prominent, a deflectable ablation catheter can be placed, with or without a guiding sheath, through the femoral vein. This catheter can be negotiated into the coronary sinus and the deflection mechanism can be used to pull down or to push up the thebesian valve, allowing easier access from above.[22] For femoral access, a minimally curved sheath such as an SR0 or SR1 (Daig) can be used, with the deflectable catheter placed initially in the right ventricle, then pulled down posteriorly with a sharp clockwise rotation, and gradually withdrawn to engage the coronary sinus.

Valves may also cover the orifice of the middle cardiac vein or posterolateral vein (Vieussens valve) (Fig. 19-21). These valves can be visualized angiographically. If they cause difficulty with engaging a ventricular vein, gentle manipulation of a deflectable catheter usually yields the best results.

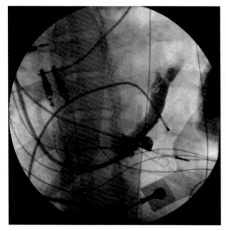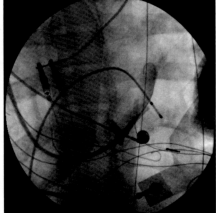

Figure 19. Angiographic frames showing a prominent valve at the junction of the coronary sinus and posterolateral vein. Note in the right frame a guidewire advance attempting to prolapse beyond the valve.

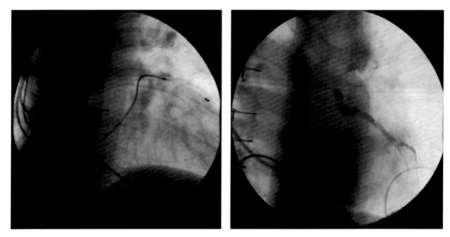

Figure 20. Multiple valves in a posterolateral vein can be visualized with angiography (right). It may be difficult to advance guidewires or small French leads beyond these valves. Larger and less pliable leads can be used in these circumstances (left).

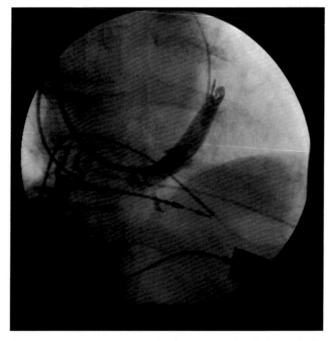

Figure 21. Coronary venous angiography showing near total occlusion at the junction of the coronary sinus and great cardiac vein.

Abnormalities of the Coronary Sinus—Coronary Sinus Stenosis, Extreme Tortuosity of the Coronary Sinus, Congenital Anomalies

Discrete coronary stenosis is rare. On angiography, the appearance of coronary sinus stenosis is often the result of right atrial musculature extending into the coronary sinus (Fig. 22).[23] Repeating angiography or waiting 5 to 10 minutes before again attempting to enter the coronary sinus may show that segmental spasm has resolved. When true coronary sinus stenosis is seen, the segment can be managed by angioplasty with low-pressure balloons and the coronary sinus can be cannulated successfully.[24] When extreme tortuosity is diagnosed with right atrial angiography, coronary arteriography, or ultrasonography, a soft wire such as an angled Glide wire should be used first to negotiate the curvature and the guiding sheath should be placed only at the ostium of the coronary sinus (Fig. 23). No attempt should be made to subselect or to advance sheaths deep into a tortuous coronary sinus (Fig. 24-26).

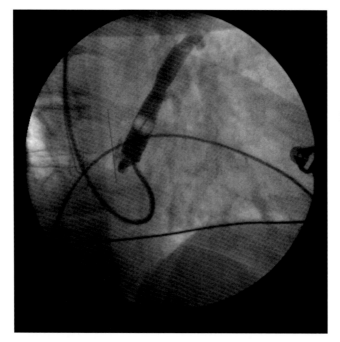

Figure 22. Backwash of contrast during coronary sinus angiography shows marked narrowing at the ostium of the coronary sinus because of a near circumferential thebesian valve. Cannulation of the vein can be accomplished with either deflectable catheters or guidewires kept close to the intra-atrial septum and entering near the roof of the coronary sinus at the ostium (see text).

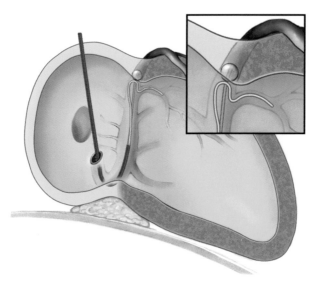

Figure 23. Posterior veins or, occasionally, a bifurcating middle cardiac vein with an acute or tortuous takeoff can be challenging for lead implantation. One approach is to use deflectable catheters and subselect the vein as described in the text. Another approach, illustrated in this figure, is to use an occlusion balloon distal to the takeoff of the branch of interest. Passing the guidewire or a small French pacing lead with the balloon deflated can help angulate or force the wire to engage the midportion of the desired vein.

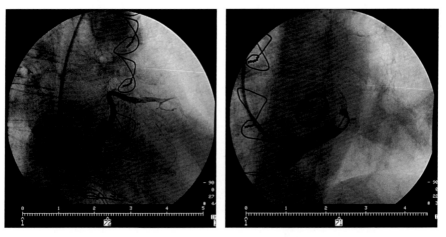

Figure 24. Angiographic images in the right and left anterior oblique projections showing an abrupt decrease in the lumen size at the junction of the coronary sinus and great cardiac vein. Although coronary sinus dissections may have this appearance, the abnormality in this patient was probably related to mitral valve surgery.

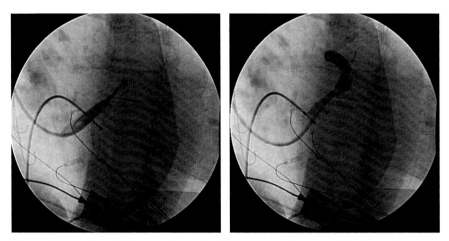

Figure 25. Angiographic images in a patient with coronary sinus stenosis. No previous instrumentation or surgical procedures had been performed on this patient. A diffuse narrowing in the mid portion of the coronary sinus was noted on angiography (left). Low-pressure balloon dilation was performed and an adequate lumen size was obtained that facilitated lead placement (right).

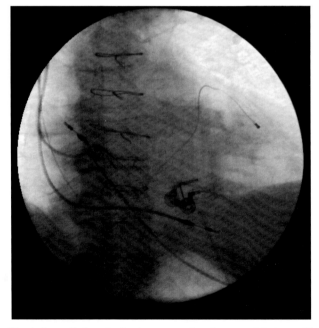

Figure 26. After balloon dilation, the lead was negotiated successfully to a mid ventricular position in the lateral wall of the left ventricle.

Complete Occlusion of the Coronary Sinus

Complete occlusion of the coronary sinus is extremely rare. On coronary arteriography or right atrial angiography, the appearance of a complete valve or occlusion at the ostium of the coronary sinus is usually the result of a prominent thebesian valve that is fenestrated (Fig. 27-29).[25] We have observed one instance of complete occlusion

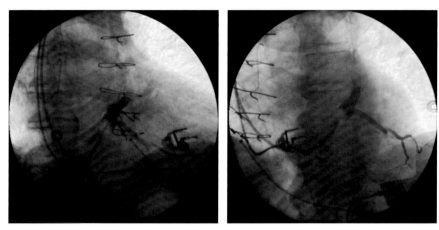

Figure 27. Angiography showing an abrupt termination of the coronary sinus. More proximal venography demonstrated a posterior and lateral vein takeoff proximal to the obstruction. This vein was used for lead placement. This patient had previously had radiofrequency ablation within the coronary sinus for Wolff-Parkinson-White syndrome.

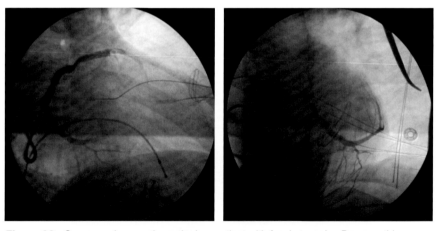

Figure 28. Coronary sinus angiography in a patient with focal stenosis. Because this patient had extensive collaterals to the lateral circulation via a posterior ventricular vein whose ostium was proximal to the stenosis, angioplasty was not necessary. The lead was manipulated via the collaterals to an adequate position in the lateral ventricular wall.

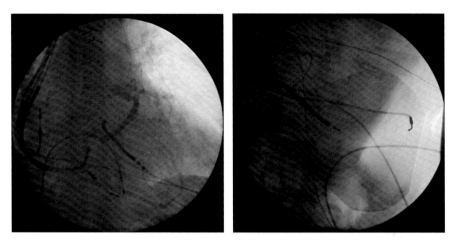

Figure 29. Fluoroscopic images showing lead placement via collaterals to the lateral wall.

at the ostium of the coronary sinus in a patient who previously had a radiofrequency ablation procedure. In these instances, the coronary venous flow reaches either the right atrium or the right ventricle through collateral atrial or ventricular thebesian veins. A similar drainage to a ventricular location can also be seen after certain surgical corrections of congenital anomalies. In these cases, right atrial angiography with a pigtail catheter placed in the right atrium or coronary arteriography is critical for diagnosing the cause of the difficulty. If a prominent atrial vein is seen draining coronary sinus blood, a technique similar to that for managing a prominent inferior thebesian valve can be used. A straight sheath and a deflectable catheter are placed along the septum in the region of the fossa ovalis and the atrial vein is cannulated. The sheath can be placed in the atrial vein and the lead deployed. When single or multiple ventricular veins are seen collateralizing the proximal occlusion, a deflectable catheter capable of delivering intravenous contrast (Irvine Biomedical) can be used to gently engage one of these vessels.[24] The sheath usually cannot be advanced through these vessels and is best placed at the ostium of the ventricular collateral. An over-the-wire left ventricular lead can be negotiated back to the main body of the coronary sinus. Care must be taken because thebesian vessels may anastomose with similar vessels in the interventricular septum and drain the left ventricle. In this instance, the lead may inadvertently be left endocardially in the left ventricle.

Placement of a coronary venous lead may also be hampered by a focal narrowing within the great cardiac vein (Fig. 30).

Complications Associated With Coronary Sinus Cannulation

Dissection of the coronary sinus may occur when engaging the coronary sinus or

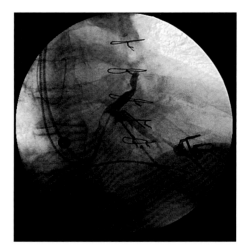

Figure 30. Coronary sinus angiography demonstrating focal narrowing in the great cardiac vein. Such narrowing appears to be more common in patients who have had valvular or bypass surgery.

attempting to advance the sheath into the coronary sinus.[26] Angiography from the coronary sinus will show staining of the coronary sinus musculature, the coronary sinus wall, or occasionally extensive staining of the entire coronary venous tree. Mild localized dissections of the coronary sinus are probably inconsequential, and the procedure can be performed in the usual fashion. More extensive dissections lead to closure of the coronary venous system, precluding placement of the lead (Fig. 31 and 32).[24] The natural history of these occlusions is not known. When a coronary sinus dissection is diagnosed, the pericardium should be carefully examined fluoroscopically during injection of dye.[27] If no perforation is seen, a soft wire such as a Glide wire can be advanced after the sheath is pulled back to the ostium and negotiated beyond the dissection. Over this wire, a multipurpose angiographic sheath can be advanced beyond the dissection. A soft wire over which the left ventricular lead can be advanced should first be advanced through the multipurpose sheath to a distal portion of the ventricular vein. The multipurpose sheath can be removed and the lead advanced over this wire and beyond the dissection. True coronary sinus perforations are recognized by the extravasation of contrast dye injected in the coronary sinus. Also, the clinical or echocardiographic features of pericardial effusion are usually seen. Tamponade is unusual because of the low-flow coronary venous system.[28,29] However, if a sheath is advanced inadvertently through a perforated segment, life-threatening tamponade may occur. Coronary sinus perforations may also occur into the posteroseptal space, the oblique sinus behind the left atrium, or the mediastinum. Computed tomographic scanning with the use of contrast may be required to monitor the extent of bleeding.[30]

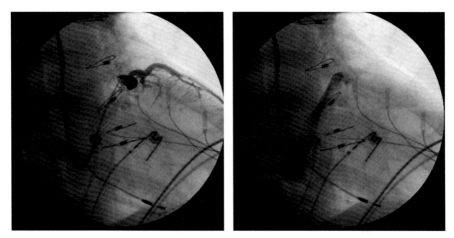

Figure 31. Coronary sinus angiogram in a patient with highly tortuous distal great cardiac vein and ventricular veins. Forceful injection to adequately visualize the distal veins resulted in a pericardial blush (staining), which can result from coronary sinus dissection, pericardial infiltration, or contrast within the thebesian vein network. Cine fluoroscopy will show characteristic annular movement with coronary sinus dissection but movement with the cardiac silhouette in pericardial and intramyocardial staining.

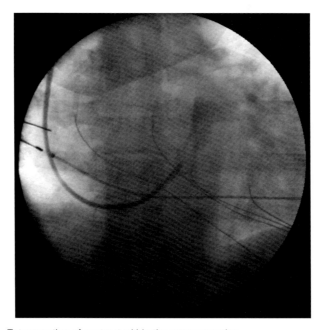

Figure 32. Extravasation of contrast within the coronary veins.

Left Ventricular Lead Deployment

After the coronary sinus has been cannulated, the guiding sheath is used to advance the left ventricular pacing lead through the sinus into a ventricular vein. Acute intra-operative epicardial lead data suggest that maximal benefit is achieved with a mid-lateral positioning of the lead, but currently no long-term data are available about the ideal location of the lead.[31,32] Thus, lead stability and obtaining sufficient separation from the right ventricular lead are the primary considerations in choosing the left ventricular pacing site. Over-the-wire left ventricular pacing leads have been a major advance in increasing the ease of selecting ventricular venous pacing sites.[33]

General Considerations

Both stylet-driven and over-the-wire leads are available for clinical use. Operators are usually familiar with stylet-driven leads. The stylet can be preformed to various curvatures. Also, retracting and inserting the stylet at the tip of the lead can change the angulation at the tip so the lead can be maneuvered into a ventricular venous branch. In most cases, over-the-wire leads are preferable because it is easier to negotiate more distal locations in the venous system. If the over-the-wire system is used, the wire is first inserted through the sheath and placed in the vein of interest, and then the lead is loaded on the over-the-wire system and advanced into the vein (Fig. 33). Typically, small French-size leads are preferred so that the lead tip can be left in a subbranch or tributary of a major ventricular vein, aiding stability. In some instances, however, the coronary sinus and ventricular veins may be grossly dilated and the small French-size lead cannot make adequate contact with the myocardial surface. In this case, larger stylet-driven leads can be used and placed relatively more proximally in the coronary venous system to make better contact. Similarly, larger stylet-driven leads may be useful when pacing thresholds are poor in the mid and distal portions of the ventricle or when a lead needs to be placed in the proximal venous system, where venous diameter is large and smaller leads may not make adequate contact with the myocardium. Various lengths of leads are available. The author prefers to use relatively long lengths (approximately 85 cm) because they afford the option of cannulating secondary branches, distal branches, and anasto-motic branches.[34] Furthermore, in greatly enlarged hearts, the anterior interven-tricular vein occasionally cannot be reached with standard-length leads (Fig. 34).

Techniques to Ensure Lead Stability

When the left ventricular lead is advanced, gentle pressure should cause mild buckling in the coronary sinus and proximal ventricular vein so that the lead conforms to the curvature of the venous system. Another technique to enhance stability is to advance the lead through a main ventricular venous branch, for example, the posterolateral vein, and use the wire to subselect a tributary and

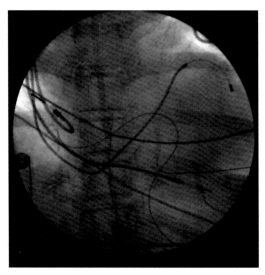

Figure 33. Fluoroscopy of a stylet-driven pacing lead in a lateral cardiac vein. Stylet-driven leads are more difficult to manipulate than the commonly used over-the-wire pacing leads; however, because of their larger diameter, they can be useful when placing leads in the proximal portion of dilated cardiac veins (see text).

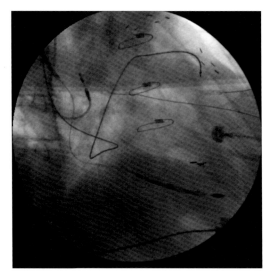

Figure 34. Fluoroscopic image of an over-the-wire lead placed in a lateral branch of the anterior interventricular vein. Collaterals or anastomotic branches exist between the anterior and lateral venous systems. Longer leads may be required to navigate through these collaterals to eventually achieve a location in the mid-lateral left ventricular wall.

advance this to a yet secondary tributary that is in parallel with the primary vein. This U-shaped placement usually is highly resistant to dislodgement during removal of the sheath. Care should be taken to prevent excess slack or buckling proximal to the ostium of the coronary sinus. After the sheath has been removed, the tricuspid annular region should be inspected carefully. If the lead prolapses beyond the tricuspid valve into the right ventricle, a soft stylet should be inserted and the slack removed. Excess slack within a large dilated coronary sinus may cause coiling or looping of the lead in the coronary sinus. In our experience at Mayo Clinic, this has not affected lead stability and we have elected to leave the loop within the coronary sinus. Occasionally, excessive slack caus-es prolapse of the proximal portion of the lead into the inferior vena cava. It is probably best to pull back on the lead to minimize the slack (Fig. 35).

If the coronary venous system is very large (dilated and nearly variceal), obtaining contact and adequate wedging is a problem with even larger leads.[35,36] To overcome this challenge, two techniques may be used. 1) The over-the-wire lead system can be advanced through the large venous system from, for example, the posterolateral vein all the way to the apex and then advanced through either the anterior interventricular vein or middle cardiac vein to a more proximal location,

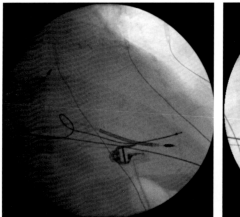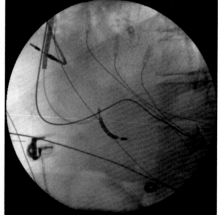

Figure 35. Fluoroscopic images of over-the-wire leads placed in the region of the lateral left ventricle. Various techniques can be used to enhance lead stability. Left, Note a loop within the proximal dilated coronary veins. Loops may enhance stability in certain venous locations. Respiratory maneuvers and patient repositioning should be performed before closure. Right, An ideal positioning of the lead tip is shown. The tip has been advanced through a main coronary vein into a subsidiary branch that is parallel with this vein. This type of positioning is particularly useful in very dilated hearts and when dislodgement occurs repeatedly within the main vein.

where the lead can be placed in a smaller venous tributary. 2) The left ventricular lead is purposely curled on itself and advanced as a loop into the dilated venous system. To do this, the wire is first advanced to engage a venous branch. Thus engaged, the lead is continuously pushed until the body of the lead begins to pro-lapse as a loop into the great cardiac vein. The wire is then retracted and the lead is advanced as a loop into another venous branch. Advancing the lead with this loop sometimes affords better myocardial contact and adequate thresholds when previous maneuvers were unsuccessful. This same maneuver can also be helpful in avoiding diaphragmatic stimulation when a proximal posterolateral or middle cardiac vein is used. When advanced as a loop, the tip of the lead can be manipu-lated to be oriented more toward the myocardium than the diaphragm.

Thresholds should be checked before and after the sheath has been removed. High output (at the highest output and pulse width setting) should be performed during both inspiration and expiration to check for phrenic or diaphragmatic stim-ulation. In our experience, if diaphragmatic stimulation occurs, it is preferable to obtain access in a different venous branch than to attempt repositioning the lead in the same vein, because diaphragmatic stimulation may occur subacutely with movement or change in respiration.

Deployment in the Middle Cardiac Vein

If it is not possible to place the guiding sheath in the middle cardiac vein, the fol-lowing technique can be performed (Fig. 36). (A similar technique can be used also to cannulate posterolateral and lateral veins when standard techniques have failed.) An occlusive balloon, as used for angiography, is advanced beyond the orifice of the middle cardiac vein (or vein of interest). The wire for the over-the-wire pacing lead is advanced alongside the balloon in the sheath placed at the ostium of the coronary sinus. The balloon is fully deployed distally to the orifice of the venous branch. The wire is then advanced; however, because it cannot advance beyond the balloon, it usually curls back toward the sheath. While the wire curls back toward the sheath, the angulation of the sheath can be changed slightly so that the wire will track in a ventricular direction in the RAO projection. By switching to an LAO projection, it can be ascertained whether the wire has tracked back toward the right ventricle or is in the middle cardiac vein. Next, the wire is manipulated carefully to remove excess slack and to advance it as far as possible in the middle cardiac vein (Fig. 37). The pacing lead is advanced over the wire into the vein after the balloon catheter has been removed. It is not uncommon when one tries to select the middle cardiac vein that the sheath, deflectable catheter, or wire instead cannulates the infradiaphrag-matic, or suprasplenic, vein. This vein takes the course of the middle cardiac vein and can mimic a lateral branch of the middle cardiac vein. Usually, excellent ven-tricular sensing and reasonable thresholds for pacing are achieved with a lead placed in this branch. However, diaphragmatic stimulation and lead dislodgement are

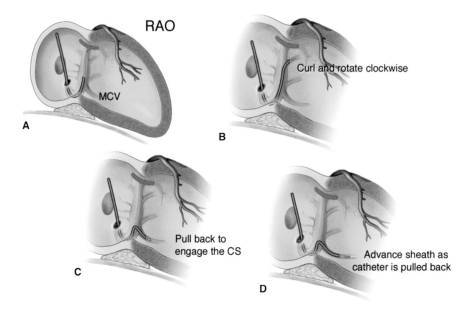

Figure 36. The technique for cannulating proximal posterior and middle cardiac vein (MCV). A, In the right anterior oblique (RAO) projection, the deflectable catheter is aimed at the posterior pericardial fat pad region. Counterclockwise torque is applied to engage the coronary sinus (CS), as previously described. B, After the catheter is in the main body of the coronary sinus, a bend is placed to point the tip in a ventricular direction in the RAO projection. With this orientation, clockwise torque is applied. C, With clockwise torque being applied, the catheter is drawn back toward the ostium where posterior veins and the middle cardiac vein will be engaged. D, The catheter is advanced into the vein, and with gentle to-and-fro manipulation, the sheath is used to subselect this vein.

frequent with leads placed in this vein. A simple maneuver with deep inspiration will clarify that the lead and vein are below the diaphragm.

Sheath Removal

After the lead has been placed satisfactorily and preliminary thresholds have been checked to ensure local ventricular capture and to exclude extracardiac stimulation, the guiding sheath needs to be removed. Several methods are available for removing the sheath, including peel-away type sheaths and cutting-away systems. Also, with certain combinations of lead and sheath, the sheath can be pulled over the lead. Regardless of the system used, certain principles need to be followed. A stylet should be reintroduced into the lead before the sheath is removed. Depending on the lead system, the stylet may be introduced all the way

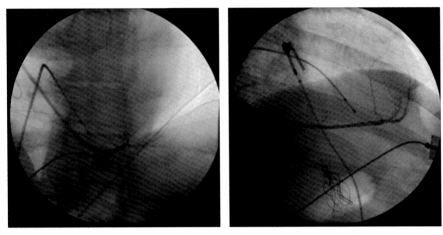

Figure 37. Selective angiography of a subselected middle cardiac vein showing numerous lateral branches that will allow lead placement at the lateral ventricular wall.

to the tip of the lead or into the main body of the coronary sinus. Despite these variations, the stylet should be of medium stiffness (in most cases) and placed at least 1 cm into the coronary sinus and preferably in the great cardiac vein. If the stylet is placed too close to the coronary sinus or in the right atrium, pulling back on the sheath may cause excessive inferior force and dislodge the lead. Whether the sheath is cut away, peeled away, or removed over the lead, the lead should be held firmly in place while the sheath is removed. In the case of the cut-away system, the cutting blade should be secured to the lead and the blade and lead held firmly onto the patient with one hand. The sheath should be pulled back against the blade and care taken not to change the existing rotational torque on the sheath. In other words, the sheath should be pulled back in the angle in which it lays and not be maneuvered to suit the operator. This is to avoid dislodging the lead as the sheath is cut back. The movement should be smooth and fluid, and the hand that stabilizes the lead should not be moved. Similarly, with peel-away or over-the-lead removal, the hand that stabilizes the lead should not move, and the tendency to push the lead further into the body should be resisted. After the sheath has been removed, the lead is secured to its sleeve and the sleeve to the underlying muscle. Most operators remove the stylet for suturing the lead and introduce the stylet up to the junction of the superior vena cava and right atrium before manipulating other leads. Fluoroscopy should be performed after the stylet has been removed and the lead has been secured to ensure there is no excess slack, specifically slack that causes the body of the lead to prolapse into the right ventricle.

Miscellaneous Challenges to Effective Cannulation and Lead Deployment in the Coronary Sinus

Congenital anomalies, particularly those associated with malposition of the heart (situs inversus, dextrocardia, and dextroversion) can make coronary sinus cannulation and lead deployment challenging. The operator must study the data available for the patient, including transesophageal echocardiograms, chest radiographs, and angiograms (if these studies have been performed in the patient). Generally, neutral sheaths, either straight or with minimal curvature, and deflectable catheters capable of recording electrograms can be useful in overcoming some of the challenges. Intracardiac ultrasonography, particularly to visualize the tricuspid valve and fossa ovalis, may provide useful landmarks for attempts at cannulating the coronary sinus. An exception to the rule that a congenital anomaly makes placing a left ventricular lead more difficult is the anomaly with a persistent left superior vena cava (Fig. 38 and 39). In these patients, it can be easier to place a left ventricular lead (although it is less stable) than a right ventricular lead. Following the natural vertical angle of the persistent left superior vena cava ventricularly in the RAO projection results in cannulation of the posterolateral vein or, less commonly, a lateral coronary vein. In these patients, it occasionally can be difficult to deploy the right ventricular lead, especially when no connections to the right superior vena cava are present. Here, the guiding system typically used for placing the left ventricular lead can be used to place smaller French-size pacing leads into the right ventricle after a deflectable

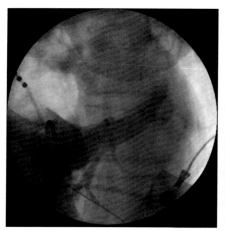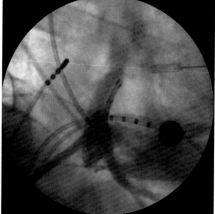

Figure 38. Coronary sinus angiography showing a large aneurysmal coronary sinus. Note the multipolar catheter placed in the His bundle region showing the extent of the enlargement of the coronary sinus ostium. A persistent left superior vena cava should be excluded and extra precautions should be taken to ensure lead stability (see text).

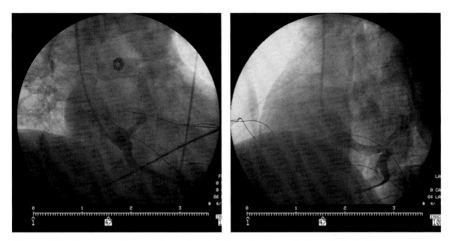

Figure 39. Coronary sinus angiography showing a large posterior vein but with a narrow neck. Two kinds of problems may arise with lead placement in such cases. One, cannulating the vein itself can be difficult because of the narrow neck. Two, after the lead is placed in a large vein, contact with the myocardium may not be adequate. Either curling the lead on itself or subselecting a branch or placing a larger diameter lead may be required for good myocardial contact.

catheter allows the sheath to be placed within the right ventricular chamber. The sheath can then be peeled away or cut away and an adequate result obtained. If a persistent left superior vena cava is present in combination with adequate connections to the right superior vena cava, the left ventricular lead can be placed through the left superior vena cava and the right ventricular lead through the right superior vena cava. In patients with a mechanical prosthetic tricuspid valve in place, epicardial pacing via thoracotomy is clearly preferred. If epicardial pacing cannot be accomplished safely, a coronary sinus pacing lead can be placed. To avoid entrapment of the leads across the tricuspid valve, intracardiac ultrasonography or transesophageal echocardiography should be used throughout the procedure to visualize the tricuspid valve and extreme caution should be used in manipulating the leads.

Summary

Multiple approaches can be used to cannulate the coronary sinus and deploy a left ventricular lead. The choice of a particular approach depends on the training and background of the operator and the resources available. Also, it is desirable to know several solutions to any problem that may develop. No single sheath, curvature, deflectable catheter, wire, or technique is ideally suited for all patients. Although most operators become familiar with a particular set of techniques, they should be willing to try another technique that may be helpful in a difficult case.

The following algorithmic approach is provided to help operators troubleshoot a difficult case. In most instances, the use of fluoroscopy and manipulation of the guide wire or deflectable catheter will engage the coronary sinus and allow effective deployment of the sheath. However, if this is difficult, the catheter should be placed in the ventricle and gradually pulled back while counterclockwise torque is applied to engage the coronary sinus. This is effective in some instances of a superior thebesian valve, prominent eustachian ridge, or reconstituted coronary sinus via ventricular veins. Should this maneuver not be effective, an attempt should be made to have a straight sheath with a deflectable catheter curve into the fossa ovalis or region of the His bundle and prolapse inferiorly along the septum. This technique is useful in patients with a large right atrium and inferior thebesian valve or an occluded coronary sinus that reconstitutes via an atrial vein. Should this fail and the heart is known to be asymmetrically and grossly enlarged, the right ventricular lead should be placed in the apex or at the site of the His bundle, which is found by mapping the typical His bundle potential. This helps define the ideal LAO projection. Once this is accomplished, the maneuvers described above can be attempted again. Should this not be successful, right atrial angiography, intracardiac ultrasonography, transesophageal echocardiography, or coronary arteriography can be performed to identify and define the coronary sinus. After the sheath has been effectively placed, the wire can be fed into the lead in an over-the-wire system. With the wire pulled back into the lead, the lead can first be advanced to determine if a lateral ventricular vein has been entered (Fig. 40 and 41). If not or if the lead does not progress to at least the mid portion of the ventricle, the wire is used to help select and obtain a more distal location in a lateral ventricular vein. If the lateral vein cannot be negotiated or the thresholds are poor at that location, the anterior interventricular vein or the middle cardiac vein can be cannulated, as outlined above. The sheath is then removed, taking care to not move the lead.

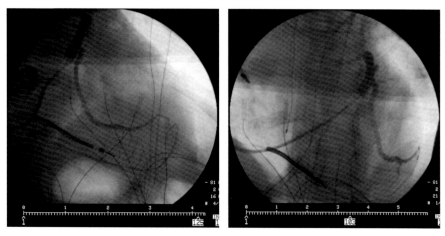

Figure 40. Coronary sinus angiography showing large anastomotic veins between the inferior and lateral coronary venous systems. Some studies have indicated that optimal lead location is in the lateral wall of the ventricle. When confronted with difficulty in cannulating the lateral vein, collaterals from other venous drainage sources can be used to place a lead in the lateral wall.

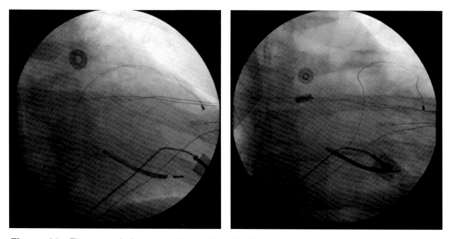

Figure 41. Fluoroscopic images in the right and left anterior projections showing lead placement in the mid-lateral wall of the left ventricle by entering through an anterior intraventricular vein and subselecting one of its lateral branches.

References

1. Cazeau S, Leclercq C, Lavergne T, Walker S, Varma C, Linde C, et al., for the Multisite Stimulation in Cardiomyopathies (MUSTIC) Study Investigators. Effects of multisite biventricular pacing in patients with heart failure and intraventricular conduction delay. N Engl J Med 2001;344:873-80.
2. Abraham WT. Cardiac resynchronization therapy for heart failure: biventricular pacing and beyond. Curr Opin Cardiol 2002;17:346-52.
3. Leclercq C, Walker S, Linde C, Clementy J, Marshall AJ, Ritter P, et al. Comparative effects of permanent biventricular and right-univentricular pacing in heart failure patients with chronic atrial fibrillation. Eur Heart J 2002;23:1780-7.
4. Maros TN, Racz L, Plugor S, Maros TG. Contributions to the morphology of the human coronary sinus. Anat Anz 1983;154:133-44.
5. Gerber TC, Kantor B, Keelan PC, Hayes DL, Schwartz RS, Holmes DR. The coronary venous system: an alternate portal to the myocardium for diagnostic and therapeutic procedures in invasive cardiology. Curr Interv Cardiol Rep 2000;2:27-37.
6. Gerber TC, Sheedy PF, Bell MR, Hayes DL, Rumberger JA, Behrenbeck T, et al. Evaluation of the coronary venous system using electron beam computed tomography. Int J Cardiovasc Imaging 2001;17:65-75.
7. Gilard M, Mansourati J, Etienne Y, Larlet JM, Truong B, Boschat J, et al. Angiographic anatomy of the coronary sinus and its tributaries. Pacing Clin Electrophysiol 1998;21:2280-4.
8. Giudici M, Winston S, Kappler J, Shinn T, Singer I, Scheiner A, et al. Mapping the coronary sinus and great cardiac vein. Pacing Clin Electrophysiol 2002;25:414-9.
9. Ortale JR, Gabriel EA, Iost C, Marquez CQ. The anatomy of the coronary sinus and its tributaries. Surg Radiol Anat 2001;23:15-21.
10. Potkin BN, Roberts WC. Size of coronary sinus at necropsy in subjects without cardiac disease and in patients with various cardiac conditions. Am J Cardiol 1987;60:1418-21.
11. Meisel E, Pfeiffer D, Engelmann L, Tebbenjohanns J, Schubert B, Hahn S, et al. Investigation of coronary venous anatomy by retrograde venography in patients with malignant ventricular tachycardia. Circulation 2001;104:442-7.
12. Melo WD, Prudencio LA, Kusnir CE, Pereira AL, Marques V, Vieira MC, et al. Angiography of the coronary venous system: use in clinical electrophysiology [Portuguese]. Arq Bras Cardiol 1998;70:409-13.
13. Grzybiak M. Morphology of the coronary sinus and contemporary cardiac electrophysiology. Folia Morphol (Warsz) 1996;55:272-3.
14. Meinertz T. A study of coronary sinus (v. cava cran. sin.), the middle cardiac vein and the aortic arch as well as ductus (lig.) Botalli in a number of mammal hearts [German]. Gegenbaurs Morphol Jahrb 1966;109:473-500.
15. Duda B, Grzybiak M. Main tributaries of the coronary sinus in the adult human heart. Folia Morphol (Warsz) 1998;57:363-9.
16. Asirvatham S, Packer DL. Evidence of electrical conduction within the coronary sinus musculature by non-contact mapping [abstract]. Circulation 1999;100 Suppl 1:I-850.
17. Maurer G, Punzengruber C, Haendchen RV, Torres MA, Heublein B, Meerbaum S, et al. Retrograde coronary venous contrast echocardiography: assessment of shunting and delineation of regional myocardium in the normal and ischemic canine heart. J Am Coll Cardiol 1984;4:577-86.
18. D'Cruz IA, Shala MB, Johns C. Echocardiography of the coronary sinus in adults. Clin Cardiol 2000;23:149-54.

19. von Ludinghausen M. Clinical anatomy of cardiac veins, Vv. cardiacae. Surg Radiol Anat 1987;9:159-68.
20. Dobosz PM, Kolesnik A, Aleksandrowicz R, Ciszek B. Anatomy of the valve of the coronary (Thebesian valve). Clin Anat 1995;8:438-9.
21. Duda B, Grzybiak M. Variability of valve configuration in the lumen of the coronary sinus in the adult human hearts. Folia Morphol (Warsz) 2000;59:207-9.
22. Ansari A. Anatomy and clinical significance of ventricular Thebesian veins. Clin Anat 2001;14:102-10.
23. Zanoschi C. Malformations of the coronary sinus [Romanian]. Rev Med Chir Soc Med Nat Iasi 1986;90:749-52.
24. Sandler DA, Feigenblum DY, Bernstein NE, Holmes DS, Chinitz LA. Cardiac vein angioplasty for biventricular pacing. Pacing Clin Electrophysiol 2002;25:1788-9.
25. Kuta W, Grzybiak M, Nowicka E. The valve of the coronary sinus (Thebasian) in adult human hearts. Folia Morphol (Warsz) 2000;58:263-74.
26. Alonso C, Leclercq C, d'Allonnes FR, Pavin D, Victor F, Mabo P, et al. Six year experience of transvenous left ventricular lead implantation for permanent biventricular pacing in patients with advanced heart failure: technical aspects. Heart 2001;86:405-10.
27. Walker S, Levy T, Paul VE. Dissection of the coronary sinus secondary to pacemaker lead manipluation. Pacing Clin Electrophysiol 2000;23:541-3.
28. Asirvatham S, Johnson SB, Seward JB, Packer DL. Utility of intracardiac ultrasound (ICUS) Doppler hemodynamics with tandem balloon catheter pulmonary venous ablation [abstract]. J Am Soc Echocardiogr 1999;12:410.
29. Asirvatham S, Johnson SB, Packer DL. Utility of intracardiac ultrasound (ICUS) in guiding circumferential pulmonary venous ablation with a tandem balloon catheter [abstract]. Pacing Clin Electrophysiol 1999;22:822.
30. Wahl MR, Roman-Gonzalez J, Asirvatham S, Johnson SB, Camp JJ, Robb RA, et al. Spatial fusion of ultrasound with computed tomographic imaging of the heart to facilitate 3D mapping [abstract]. Pacing Clin Electrophysiol 2000;23:626.
31. Auricchio A, Stellbrink C, Sack S, Block M, Vogt J, Bakker P, et al. The Pacing Therapies for Congestive Heart Failure (PATH-CHF) study: rationale, design, and endpoints of a prospective randomized multicenter study. Am J Cardiol 1999;83:130D-5D.
32. Bordachar P, Garrigue S, Reuter S, Hocini M, Kobeissi A, Gaggini G, et al. Hemodynamic assessment of right, left, and biventricular pacing by peak endocardial acceleration and echocardiography in patients with end-stage heart failure. Pacing Clin Electrophysiol 2000;23:1726-30.
33. Achtelik M, Bocchiardo M, Trappe H-J, Gaita F, Lozano I, Niazi I, et al., the VENTAK CHF/CONTAK CD Clinical Investigation Study Group. Performance of a new steroid-eluting coronary sinus lead designed for left ventricular pacing. Pacing Clin Electrophysiol 2000;23:1741-3.
34. Sack S, Heinzel F, Dagres N, Enger S, Auricchio A, Stellbrink C, et al. Stimulation of the left ventricle through the coronary sinus with a newly developed 'over the wire' lead system: early experiences with handling and positioning. Europace 2001;3:317-23.
35. Schaffler GJ, Groell R, Peichel KH, Rienmuller R. Imaging the coronary venous drainage system using electron-beam CT. Surg Radiol Anat 2000;22:35-9.
36. Sethna DH, Moffitt EA. An appreciation of the coronary circulation. Anesth Analg 1986;65:294-305.

CHAPTER 5

Optimization of Biventricular Devices

Samuel J. Asirvatham, MD
David L. Hayes, MD

A body of literature has established the usefulness of biventricular pacing systems in improving the quality of life of patients with heart failure.[1-3] It appears, however, that some patients do not have a response to this form of therapy. Optimal programming of the device may turn "nonresponders" into "responders" and "responders" into "better responders" to biventricular stimulation. The ideal method for optimizing existing devices is not known. Many methods have been suggested, including the use of echocardiographic, electrocardiographic (ECG), and lead position variables. Most of these recommendations are based on a particular optimization method used in a large trial that eventually showed benefit with biventricular pacing or on an entirely empiric, albeit logical, hemodynamic or echocardiographic model. The important effort of finding the ideal settings and lead position for biventricular systems is developing rapidly, but no firm conclusions can be drawn. This chapter outlines the basis for existing recommendations for optimizing biventricular systems and briefly reviews the theory and technique of the main optimization methods.

Atrioventricular Optimization

Optimizing the atrioventricular (AV) interval is, in a sense, optimizing the preload conditions for the left ventricle. The ideal mechanical timing for a pacing system to predict the optimal preload for the left ventricle often has to rely on echocardiographic or invasive hemodynamic measurements. Patients who require biventricular systems frequently have abnormal and variable intra-atrial and intraventricular conduction delays. This makes predicting left-sided AV mechanical delay difficult using right atrial pacing. Thus, the same AV interval will result in markedly varying left-sided AV mechanical intervals in different patients because of their individual amount of intra-atrial and intraventricular conduction delay. Also, the exact site of both ventricular and atrial lead placement has to be considered when optimizing AV timing. For example, a patient with an atrial lead placed on the intra-atrial septum and a left ventricular lead placed near the base of the left ventricle will have completely different AV mechanical timing than a patient with right atrial appendage pacing and left ventricular apical pacing, even though the AV interval is set similarly.

The rationale for ventricular resynchronization is primarily to normalize the ventricular activation sequence and to coordinate septal and free wall contraction, thereby improving cardiac efficiency.[4] Although this is independent of AV conduction and mechanical AV delays, an incremental benefit above that achieved with ventricular resynchronization has been demonstrated within a range of ideal AV delay.[5] Nishimura et al.[6] have demonstrated the effects of nonoptimal AV delay in heart failure. With long AV delays, there is a suboptimal contribution of atrial systole. This gives rise to diastolic mitral regurgitation and limits the diastolic filling that occurs as a result of active atrial systole. Shortening AV delay decreases the amount of diastolic mitral regurgitation and dilated cardiomyopathy, thereby decreasing pulmonary capillary wedge pressures. In contrast, an AV delay that is too short gives rise to a nonoptimal shortened AV filling period for the left ventricle and thus decreased preload and cardiac output.

Intra-atrial conduction even in the normal heart is poorly understood. The degree and extent of intra-atrial conduction delays in patients with heart failure and abnormal hearts are highly variable. In the normal state, sinus impulses from the junction of the right atrium and superior vena cava reach the left atrium primarily through the roof of the atrium (Bachmann bundle) and secondarily through the fossa ovalis and musculature of the coronary sinus.[7] Once the impulses reach the atria, a distinct sequence of activation involving predictable differences in activation of the posterior atrium, left atrial appendages, and pulmonary vein is observed. While intra-atrial conduction is occurring, conduction via the AV node to the ventricle also occurs. In patients without bundle branch block, the right and left mid endocardial surfaces of the intraventricular septum are activated nearly simultaneously. With AV pacing using a right atrial appendage lead and a right ventricular apical lead configuration, increased intra-atrial conduction delay may give rise to near simultaneous left atrial and left ventricular activation, producing the equivalent of a left-sided pacemaker syndrome. However, placement of the atrial lead in the region of the Bachmann bundle in a patient with insignificant intra-atrial conduction delay but significant conduction delay from the right ventricular pacing site to the left ventricle will cause marked prolongation of the left-sided mechanical AV interval. Intra-atrial conduction delay also affects the AV interval during atrial sensing. During atrial tracking, right atrial events are sensed after the onset of atrial depolarization. In some patients, sinus activation occurs first on the septal side of the junction of the right atrium and superior vena cava. The intra-atrial delay from this site to the right atrial appendage where the pacing lead is required may be marked. By the time the atrial event is sensed in these patients, left atrial activation may be ongoing or even completed, giving rise to a very long left atrium-to-left ventricle mechanical delay with usual AV timing.

Thus, the location of the atrial lead and the right and left ventricular leads, the magnitude and differences between intra-atrial conduction and intraventricular conduction delays, and whether atrial pacing or sensing is occurring all have effects on left atrial and ventricular mechanical intervals that are difficult to predict.[8]

Left ventricular end-diastolic pressures may change significantly with the actual AV delay, and this change is mainly independent of the site of ventricular pacing.[9] Left ventricular contractility (measured as dP/dt) is also affected by the AV delay, and this effect is incremental to the benefit seen with left ventricular-based pacing over right ventricular pacing[10] (Fig. 1). In the Pacing Therapies in Congestive Heart Failure (PATH-CHF) trial, a hemodynamic benefit, as seen with increased left ventricular maximal dP/dt and increased pulse pressure, was demonstrated with either left ventricular or biventricular pacing in comparison with right ventricular-based

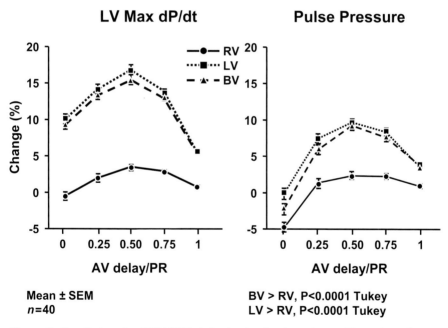

Figure 1. Results from the PATH-CHF study showing the dependence of hemodynamic response to biventricular pacing on the programmed atrioventricular (AV) delay. Expressed as a percentage of the baseline PR interval, very short and prolonged AV delay-to-PR ratios show a decrease in the LV dP/dt and pulse pressure benefit seen with biventricular (BV) and left ventricular (LV) pacing. RV, right ventricle. (From Auricchio A, Stellbrink C, Sack S, Block M, Vogt J, Bakker P, et al. Long-term clinical effect of hemodynamically optimized cardiac resynchronization therapy in patients with heart failure and ventricular conduction delay. J Am Coll Cardiol 2002;39:2026-33. By permission of the American College of Cardiology.)

pacing. However, the effect was seen best at AV delays between 25% and 75% of the intrinsic PR interval.[5] Butter et al.[11] also showed a benefit of left ventricular free-wall pacing in comparison with an anterior site in the left ventricle when measuring a percentage increase in dP/dt. This effect was also optimal at AV delays between 50 and 100 milliseconds, and prolongation of the AV delay showed a decrease in this beneficial effect on contractility regardless of the site of pacing.

Principles of Echocardiographic AV Optimization

The AV or PR interval usually is measured either from the pacemaker spike in the atrium to the ventricle or from the start of the P wave to the beginning of the QRS complex. As mentioned above, however, the mechanically relevant AV interval is the time between mechanical atrial contraction and ventricular contraction. The echocardiographic measure most useful in studying the filling characteristics of the left ventricle is mitral valve inflow Doppler velocity. The mitral valve inflow pattern in sinus rhythm is biphasic. Distinct filling waves can be recognized (Fig. 2 and 3). The first is the early filling wave (E wave). This represents blood flow into the

- **Optimized AV delay (AV_{opt}) is calculated from the formula below**

- **End of diastolic filling coincides with beginning of systole**

- **Results in**

    E- and A-wave separation

    Maximized LV DFT

$$AV_{opt} = AV_{short} + d$$
$$\text{where}$$
$$d = (AV_{long} - AV_{short}) - (QA_{pre} - QA_{spont})$$

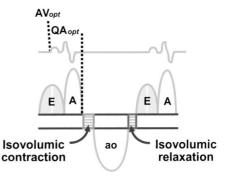

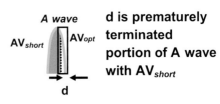

d is prematurely terminated portion of A wave with AV_{short}

Figure 2. Ritter method for optimizing atrioventricular (AV) delay (see text). ao, aortic outflow; DFT, diastolic filling time; LV, left ventricular. (Data from Ritter P, Dib J-C, Mahaux V, Lelièvre T, Soyeur D, Lavergne T, et al. New method for determining the optimal atrio-ventricular delay in patients paced in DDD mode for complete atrio-ventricular block [abstract]. Pacing Clin Electrophysiol 1995;18:855.)

- Program short **AV delay** (AV$_{short}$), **forcing closure of mitral valve (MV)**

- **Note premature shortening of A wave, reducing diastolic filling prior to aortic outflow (ao); QA$_{pre}$ is time from QRS onset to the premature end of the A wave**

- **Program** long **AV delay** (AV$_{long}$), **maintaining ventricular pre-excitation but allowing spontaneous MV closure**

- **Note delay between MV closure and start of systole marked by beginning of isovolumic contraction period;** QA$_{spont}$ **is the time from QRS onset to the spontaneous end of the A wave**

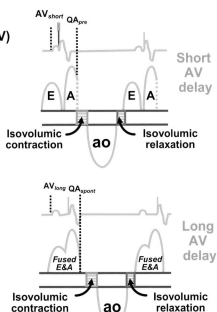

Figure 3. Ritter method for atrioventricular (AV) optimization (see text). (Data from Ritter P, Dib J-C, Mahaux V, Lelièvre T, Soyeur D, Lavergne T, et al. New method for determining the optimal atrio-ventricular delay in patients paced in DDD mode for complete atrio-ventricular block [abstract]. Pacing Clin Electrophysiol 1995;18:855.)

left ventricle during diastole. The velocity and magnitude of this flow depend primarily on the relaxation characteristics of the left ventricle. The second distinct wave is the A wave, which occurs only in sinus rhythm and is from active atrial contraction.

Because of electromechanical delays in the atrium and the ventricle, there is a distinct interval between the start of the P wave and the start of the A wave measured by mitral inflow Doppler (Fig. 4-6). In fact, the QRS complex itself is inscribed typically before the start of the A wave. When the PR interval/AV interval is short, the QRS is inscribed early and this results in aortic ejection and mitral valve closure occurring (forced by ventricular contraction) before complete inscription of the atrial and flow Doppler (truncation of the A wave). Thus, with short AV delays, diastolic flow is limited and the full benefit of atrial contraction is not obtained. This in effect is as if the patient were not in sinus rhythm and in atrial fibrillation. This is important in all patients who have congestive heart failure but especially in patients who have a severe diastolic dysfunction or relaxation abnormality. In these patients, the E wave is limited because of

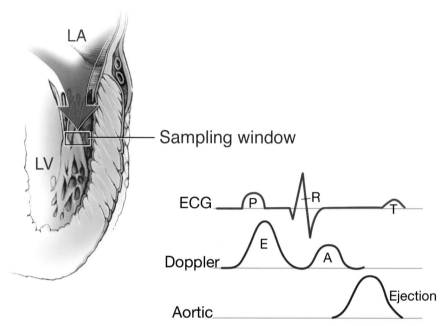

Figure 4. The principle of mitral inflow Doppler measurements to aid atrioventricular optimization. The sampling window placed at about the level of the mitral valve leaflets measures the velocity of flow from the left atrium (LA) to the left ventricle (LV). Typically, two velocities are noted: the E, or early velocity, and the A, or atrial velocity, as a result of atrial contraction. In the example shown here, the PR interval is such that complete atrial filling is noted and aortic ejection starts at about the time atrial filling is completed. This represents an ideal situation in which time is sufficient for complete atrial emptying and there is no period of diastolic mitral regurgitation.

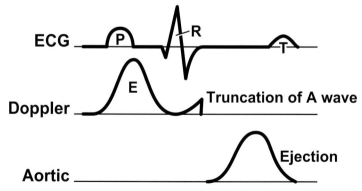

Figure 5. In this example, the PR interval or atrioventricular interval is too short. Ventricular contraction starts before atrial filling has been completed, resulting in truncation of the A wave.

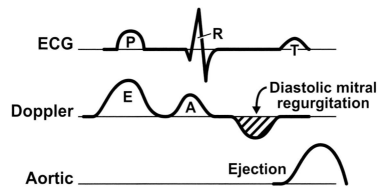

Figure 6. In this example, the PR interval or atrioventricular interval is too long. Although atrial emptying is complete, there is inordinate delay from this completion to the beginning of aortic ejection, giving rise to diastolic mitral regurgitation.

problems with ventricular relaxation and a greater portion of diastolic filling is from atrial systole and the A wave. Conversely, with a long AV interval (PR interval), the A wave is completed. However, a marked gap occurs between the end of atrial filling (A wave) and the beginning of ventricular contraction and aortic ejection (Fig. 7). During this delay, the mitral valve passively closes (soft first heart sound) and diastolic mitral regurgitation may occur. Thus, during an optimal AV interval, the atrial filling wave is completed and there is no inordinate delay between this completion and the beginning of aortic ejection.

Most methods of echocardiographic AV optimization use this principle. In one technique, the mitral inflow Doppler velocity and aortic outflow are continuously monitored echocardiographically. During this monitoring, the AV interval is set initially at about the patient's intrinsic PR interval (long AV interval). The AV interval is then progressively shortened until truncation of the atrial inflow wave is barely visible. This AV interval, with or without a small positive offset, is taken as the optimized AV interval. Using this principle that optimal AV delay results when spontaneous mitral valve closure occurs at about the same time as forced closure (ventricular contraction) and thus aortic ejection, Ritter et al.[12] have described the following method. Initially, a short AV delay (AV1) is programmed, and the interval between the onset of the QRS complex to the end of the truncated A wave (QA1) is measured. Next, a long AV delay (AV2) that maintains ventricular capture (before spontaneous AV conduction) but allows mitral valve closure before aortic ejection is measured. The interval between the start of the QRS complex and the end of the nontruncated A wave is noted (QA2). The optimal AV interval according to the Ritter calculation is AV1 + [(AV2 − AV1) − (QA1 − QA2)]. Thus, the greater the difference in the AV interval that allows complete inscription of the A wave and the short AV interval, the longer the optimal AV interval will be. On the other hand, if the difference between the start of the QRS and

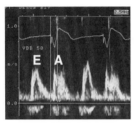

Short AV Delay
AV_{short} = 50 ms; QA_{pre} = 128 ms
(between caliper lines)

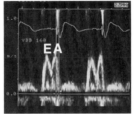

Long AV Delay
AV_{long} = 160 ms;
QA_{spont} = 48 ms

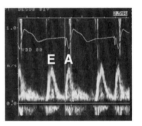

Optimized AV Delay
AV_{opt} = AV_{short} + [(AV_{long} - AV_{short}) - (QA_{pre} - QA_{spont})]

AV_{opt} = 50 + [(160 - 50) - (128 - 48)] = 80 ms

Figure 7. Echocardiographic example of atrioventricular (AV) delay optimization. With the short AV delay, truncation of the A wave is seen. Gradually lengthening the AV delay abolishes the truncation, whereas further lengthening (long AV delay) allows diastolic mitral regurgitation (see text).

the end of the A wave is small when allowing for complete AV inscription (long atrial filling), the optimal AV interval will be shorter.

Ishikawa et al.[13-15] have proposed an alternative method for AV optimization. In this relatively simpler method, a slightly prolonged AV delay is set (Fig. 8 and 9). From this number is subtracted the interval between the end of the A wave and complete closure of the mitral valve. The interval from the end of the A wave to the beginning of aortic ejection or complete closure of the mitral valve is the duration of diastolic mitral regurgitation. Thus, from a single long AV interval, the optimal AV interval can be calculated. The steps for using the Ishikawa method are to set a long AV interval and measure the mitral inflow Doppler signal. The interval between the end of the complete A wave and the beginning of aortic ejection can be measured. This measurement is subtracted from the long AV interval.

Several observations about AV optimization in the PATH-CHF study also allow for relatively simpler optimization of the AV interval. Patients with a wide QRS complex demonstrated a shorter optimal AV delay than patients with a narrow QRS complex. This is likely because intraventricular conduction delay is more prominent than interatrial conduction delay. For patients with a QRS duration greater than 150 milliseconds, the optimal average AV interval was 43% of the intrinsic AV interval. In comparison, for patients with a normal or narrower QRS complex, optimal

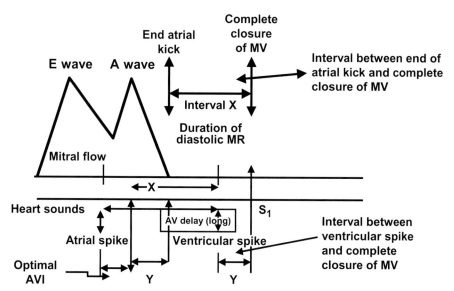

Figure 8. Ishikawa method for atrioventricular (AV) optimization (see text). AVI, AV interval; MR, mitral regurgitation; MV, mitral valve; S_1, first heart sound. (From Ishikawa T, Sumita S, Kimura K, Kikuchi M, Kosuge M, Kuji N, et al. Prediction of optimal atrioventricular delay in patients with implanted DDD pacemakers. Pacing Clin Electrophysiol 1999;22:1365-71. By permission of Blackwell Publishing.)

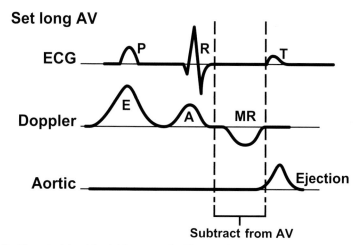

Figure 9. The principle of the Ishikawa method is to estimate the time of diastolic mitral regurgitation (MR). A long atrioventricular (AV) delay is set. The period between the end of atrial emptying and the beginning of aortic ejection is measured and subtracted from the set AV interval.

AV intervals were about 80% of the intrinsic AV interval. This, of course, will be affected by the position of the left ventricular lead. For example, if the left ventricular lead is located at a site causing early aortic ejection, then a longer AV interval will be required despite the wider QRS.

Acute hemodynamic studies have suggested that optimal ventricular contractility is further enhanced in a patient when that patient's specific AV interval is programmed. Tse et al.[16] have shown that the correlation between the impedance-measured AV interval and echocardiographic Doppler-derived AV interval is close, and the use of externally applied impedance signals is a relatively straightforward method to adjust the AV interval at the bedside. Rate-adaptive AV intervals, although of proven benefit for exercise hemodynamics in dual-chamber systems, have not been studied in biventricular systems.

Ventricular Timing Optimization (VV Optimization)

It is now possible to program an offset in the ventricle-to-ventricle (VV) timing of several biventricular systems. There is increasing need to optimize left ventricular pacing to obtain benefits beyond those obtained with cardiac resynchronization alone. Two general methods to optimize left ventricular stimulation have been proposed: spatial- and timing-related optimizations. For spatial optimization, attempts have been made to identify the ideal location of the left ventricular or right ventricular (or both) pacing leads. An early hemodynamic study suggested that the mid-lateral position in the left ventricular free wall produced the best hemodynamic benefit at rest.[17] However, because this study was performed in a relatively small number of patients and was an acute intraoperative trial, several issues remain unresolved. These include knowledge of the effect of exercise or upright posture in a nonanesthetized state. Also, it is not reasonable to postulate that this one location would be ideal for all patients, including those with lateral infarctions or poorly conducting, potentially arrhythmogenic tissue in the mid lateral wall. Attempts to individualize lead positioning have primarily used criteria derived from echocardiography and electrophysiology.

Criteria to determine the optimal location for left ventricular pacing leads have included simple QRS duration, QRS vector fusion, and combinations of these (Fig. 10 and 11). For QRS duration, various left ventricular lead positions are tried and the one that produces the shortest QRS duration is considered optimal.[18] The problem with this approach is that mechanical events do not necessarily reflect electrical events. Thus, although electrical synchronization may appear optimal, there may be areas of the ventricle with prolonged electromechanical delay that actually contract even later with the presumed electrically optimized lead position stimulation site.

Electromechanical delay or dissociation is usually insignificant in normal hearts. However, in diseased hearts, particularly ischemic ones, the time from local transmural myocardial contraction to endocardial activation can be up to 60 to 80

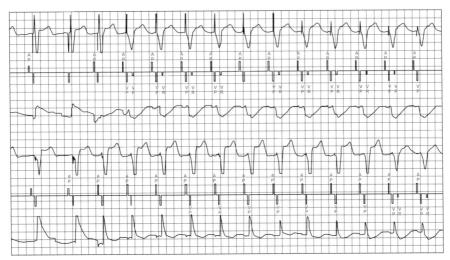

Figure 10. ECG methods for ventricle-to-ventricle optimization. A change in ECG vector and QRS duration is noted with pacing from right ventricular, left ventricular, and biventricular stimulation. Ideally with biventricular stimulation, a narrow QRS complex and a vector that is fused between pure left ventricular and right ventricular stimulation should be obtained.

milliseconds (personal observation from intracardiac echocardiographic and tissue Doppler velocity). Typically, the offsets are much greater when QRS shortening is used as an end point instead of tissue Doppler-derived criteria.

The concept of ECG vector fusion is based on the principle that a distinct vector (pattern of QRS) is associated with each pacing site. The right ventricular pacing vector and left ventricular pacing only vectors are compared (template matched with the vector resulting from biventricular pacing). Despite minimal changes in the QRS duration, if the biventricular pacing vector closely resembles the QRS complex resulting from right ventricular pacing alone, it suggests that the left ventricular pacing site makes a minimal or no contribution to global ventricular activation. This may result from exit delay from the left ventricular pacing site. In this situation, an offset can be programmed in certain devices to favor left ventricular activation (left ventricle before right ventricle by 20 to 60 milliseconds). An alternative is to reposition the left ventricular lead at implantation to a site distal to the maximal site of exit delay. This situation should be anticipated in patients with lateral wall ischemia or infarction. Here, placement of the lead either anterior or posterior to the diseased myocardial or delay site will result in both a better summed QRS vector and shortened QRS duration. This method also shares with QRS duration optimization the lack of known correlation with mechanical synchrony (see above).

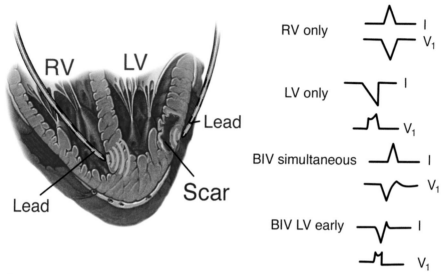

Figure 11. The principle of ECG vector fusion and its use in optimizing biventricular devices. A characteristic ECG morphology with right ventricular (RV) pacing only is noted and then with left ventricular (LV) pacing only as well. With simultaneous biventricular (BIV) stimulation, the ECG morphology is almost identical to RV pacing only. This is because of scar and tissue with delayed conduction near the LV lead. By programming an offset to stimulate the LV earlier, a true fused ECG morphology is seen.

In another method, the site of last electrical activation is noted. It is postulated that stimulation at this site of maximal delay will result in maximal synchronization. Although *electrically* this is likely to occur when pacing is targeted to the later sites of activation, *electromechanical* delay may be significant at these sites. Thus, electrical synchronization, although feasible and usually quite straightforward, lacks the appeal of mechanical optimization of ventricular lead placement.

Echocardiography for Ventricular Timing Optimization

Echocardiographic variables that have been studied to identify the best site for placing a left ventricular lead have included two-dimensional and M-mode analyses to find the sites of ventricular contraction that are delayed and occur after aortic ejection is under way. This typically involves M-mode measurement through a short-axis projection at the papillary muscle level comparing septal and free-wall contractility. The imaging plane is scanned from the apex to the base, and the site of maximal delay or dyssynchrony is targeted for lead placement. A further refinement over simple M-mode detection of delayed activation when compared with the onset of the QRS is the use of tissue Doppler velocity-derived variables. Others have used tissue

Doppler velocity imaging to measure the interval from atrial filling to the actual onset of contraction of the left ventricle. This technique, described below, may avoid the need to use surrogates for left ventricular contraction.[19]

Theoretical and Technical Basis of Tissue Velocity-Related Imaging

The usual Doppler velocity measured echocardiographically is the velocity of red blood cell flow. With appropriate changes in the filtering of frequency and amplitude, tissue velocities can be measured and displayed in color-coded and M-mode formats. Tissue Doppler velocity is the primary variable and is a measure of the actual rate of change of displacement of the myocardial fibers.[20] Currently, tissue Doppler and strain rate imaging modalities are used both experimentally and clinically to optimize biventricular pacing systems. Historically, the assessment of myocardial contractility with echocardiographic techniques has relied on visualization and quantification of myocardial thickening. The arrangement of myocardial fibers in the ventricle is complex. At various depths, the fibers are arranged either circumferentially in a spiral fashion or in a longitudinal fashion. The majority of fibers are arranged in a base-to-apex or longitudinal fashion. Thus, contraction and visualization in a longitudinal plane provide a more reliable and reproducible measure of myocardial contractility. Specifically, the epicardial fibers are arranged almost exclusively in a longitudinal, right-handed helix. The main myocardial strain vector is arranged with these longitudinal epicardial fibers. Neither two-dimensional echocardiographic nor M-mode echocardiographic assessment in short-axis projections accurately reflect this principal long-axis shortening.

Tissue Doppler velocity recorded from an apical four-chamber or long-axis view documents the velocity of contraction in this longitudinal vector (Fig. 12). The velocities are recorded relative to the transducer location, and if the transducer is located apically, shortening from apex to base will be color-coded blue and lengthening or relaxation, red. Appropriate filtering of the Doppler signal is performed to exclude blood cell velocities, which are typically about 1 m/s. Myocardial velocities are much lower, about 10 cm/s. Pulsed wave tissue Doppler can be performed to check the exact contractility in the pulse window. Multiple sampling is required for comparative purposes. Doppler data are exquisitely dependent on the frame rate. Low sampling rates/frame rates will incorrectly identify two dissimilarly contractile tissues as contracting simultaneously. Particularly with reference to optimization and biventricular systems, the temporal profile of contractility is more important than the absolute velocity of contraction, thus making frame rate even more important. Software is available with certain systems to simultaneously measure the M-mode of the tissue Doppler velocity and multiple

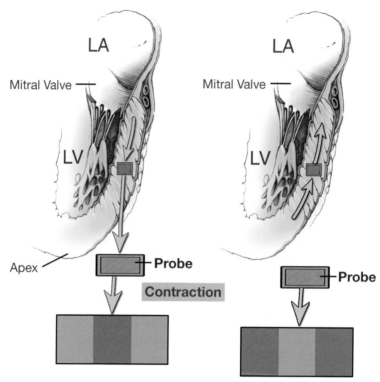

Figure 12. Doppler tissue velocity measurement. During contraction, the sampled tissue velocity has its vector toward the probe in an apical location. This results in color coding as red velocities. With relaxation, the velocity vector moves away from the probe, color coding blue. LA, left atrium; LV, left ventricle.

ventricular locations. This comparison allows identification of myocardial segments that contract later than other relatively normally functioning segments. In general cardiology, this measurement is useful for identifying ischemia, which is seen as segments that lag behind others relative to the QRS complex. With biventricular pacing, it is postulated that these lagging segments represent the most dyssynchronous portion of the ventricle and can be targeted to obtain an optimal left ventricular pacing site and to find optimal right ventricle-to-left ventricle stimulation interval timing.

A simple time integral of the velocity is the distance that the myocardial segment travels. This is a measure of the extent of contraction. Comparing this displacement or myocardial excursion at individual sites is called "tissue tracking" and is a form of parametric imaging. Thus, both velocity and displacement gradients can be calculated. The usefulness of these measurements in optimizing biventricular systems is twofold. First, the contractile distance or absolute velocity can be compared temporally to the onset of QRS during pacing. This quickly identifies segments that are late to contract. This delay in contraction may be caused by entrance delay to electrical conduction (electrical abnormality) or a delay in electromechanical coupling (ischemia). Second, using simultaneous recordings, mechanical maps can be created and readily compared with pacing from different sites, a combination of sites, and good sinus rhythm. Various global indices and scoring systems that sum overall contractility can also be used with optimizing biventricular systems to obtain the best global result.

"Strain rate" refers to the differential in velocity between two myocardial segments compared with the distance between these segments. That is,

$$\text{Strain rate} = \frac{V_1 - V_2}{d}$$

where V_1 and V_2 are the velocities of two examined segments and d is the distance between them. Thus, if two segments have highly dissimilar tissue velocities and yet are located in proximity of each other, the strain rate is high (Fig. 13). Whereas tissue velocity measures velocities relative to the transducer, strain is a measure of velocity relative to adjacent velocities. Therefore, strain is less affected by passive movement and, being more comparative, lends itself to optimizing techniques.

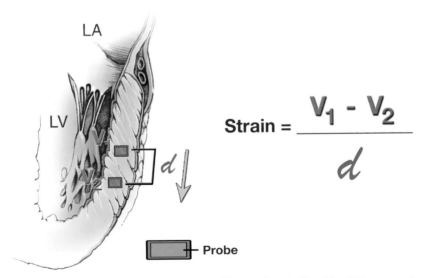

Figure 13. Strain measurements representing a difference in velocities ($V_1 - V_2$) measured over a distance (d) eliminate the effect of nonmyocardial velocities. See text for details. LA, left atrium; LV, left ventricle.

Color-coded maps for both tissue velocity and strain aid interpretation. Tissue velocity color coding is similar to the usual Doppler color coding, with blue representing velocities away from the transducer and red, velocities toward the transducer. Color coding of strain maps is different, with blue representing expansion and red representing contraction. Strain is simply a percentage change in a dimension from a resting state and represents the extent of the deformation of a particular tissue. Strain rate is the extent of this deformation over time, or the rate of deformation. Because strain rate compares two velocities, translation of velocities, for example, respiration, is factored out and, thus, strain rate represents local myocardial contractility information required when optimizing biventricular systems.[21] Harmonic tissue Doppler may be an improvement on this technique because of improved signal quality and less noise effect.

In summary, tissue velocity imaging visually displays velocity information. Tissue tracking, which is the time integral of tissue velocity, visually displays displacement of local myocardial tissue. Strain rate imaging visually displays the rate of myocardial deformation, and imaging of its time integral visually displays local myocardial deformation or contraction. One limitation of strain rate imaging is reverberation artifact. Noise from this artifact can be misjudged as dyskinesia. Because strain rate imaging involves a derivative or the rate of change of velocity signal, biases are enhanced. Both tissue velocity and strain rate imaging are angle-dependent variables.

Use of Tissue Velocity With Biventricular Devices

Although absolute velocities are a simple reflection of the health of the myocardium, the timing of the actual velocity reflects the extent of the synchrony. This can be measured in two ways: 1) timing the occurrence of peak velocity in relation to the QRS interval and 2) the relative timing of peak velocity comparing the septum and free wall or any other ventricular location. The timing from the onset of the QRS complex to mechanical activation is a reflection of electromechanical delay. Because the initial portion of the QRS complex inscribed during biventricular pacing in diseased hearts may be fragmented, isoelectric relative mechanical measurements have been used more frequently. The problem with measuring the single latest area of contraction and targeting this for lead placement is that when pacing occurs from this site, a different site may have an even more delayed mechanical activation compared with that site's activation during right ventricular pacing or sinus rhythm. In other words, the pattern of activation is changed, with early and late sites being interchanged without a net benefit. Because of this problem, scoring systems that use the extent and delay of contractility of multiple myocardial segments are summed and compared with various pacing stimulation locations. Thus, the pacing site with the best global stimulation pattern and the least intraventricular dyssynchrony and electromechanical delay is chosen in this iteration.

With the availability in some devices to program right ventricular-to-left ventricular stimulation times, similar methods have been sought to optimize the VV stimulus interval. Thus, QRS duration and QRS vector summation, decreasing the site of maximal mechanical delay, delayed tissue Doppler-derived contraction sites, and global indices improvement of tissue contraction have been studied with varying the VV interval. Tissue Doppler acceleration is derived from the tissue Doppler velocity and represents the rate at which tissue velocity changes. This parameter is less dependent on passive ventricular movement, and its timing relative to the onset of the QRS complex and tissue Doppler acceleration at other sites in the ventricle can be used in a similar manner.

The drawbacks of using tissue velocity or tissue acceleration include the following: 1) Meticulous technique to avoid artifacts of respiration and to avoid patient movement and either three-dimensional reconstruction or multiple scanning planes are required to find true late sites of activation. These late sites should be measured using multiple stimulation sites because they can vary. 2) Changes with exercise and drugs such as antiarrhythmic agents that can change the degree and dispersion of electromechanical delay must be considered as well. 3) Sites of extremely low velocity from ischemic myocardium representing poorly contractile segments may be missed completely with velocity-based imaging. 4) The frame rate, or firing rate in case of M-mode imaging, is paramount in dealing with electrical and electromechanical phenomena. The frame rate has to be sufficiently high to track electrical conduction. Electrical conduction velocities, even in diseased myocardium, are sufficiently rapid that the ideal frame rates required are in the range of 700 to 1,200 frames/s. With transthoracic imaging, one is fortunate to achieve frame rates between 100 and 150 frames/s. Thus, what is perceived as dyssynchrony between two segments is quite different when imaged with frame rates of 10 per second or 1,000 per second. With the lower frame rates, two sites may be thought to activate simultaneously when, in fact, it is an artifact of the slow change in frame rate. Intracardiac imaging using linear phased array catheters because of the proximity of the transducer to the ventricular myocardium under consideration may achieve frame rates in the range of 300 to 500 frames/s and allow better tracking of electromechanical events.

Søgaard et al.[22] examined 11 different interventricular delays in 20 patients with severe heart failure and left bundle branch block. Three-dimensional echocardiography and Doppler tissue imaging were performed before and after implantation and reexamination at 3 months. Although simultaneous cardiac resynchronization decreased the extent of myocardium that displayed delayed longitudinal contraction and improved left ventricular ejection fraction, there was an incremental benefit with sequential cardiac resynchronization. Three-dimensional echocardiography was performed during end-expiratory apnea with 1-minute breath holding using an ECG-triggered coaxial rotation from an apical transthoracic window. Tissue Doppler recordings were acquired as digital loops in end-expiratory apnea during one heartbeat in the apical four-chamber, two-chamber, and long-axis views. Typical frame rates obtained were between 100 and 135 frames/s. A 16-segment left ventricular model was applied to the transthoracic images. The global systolic contraction amplitude is calculated as the average shortening amplitude of all 16 segments. Optimal interventricular delay programming of the pacemaker was identified in each patient by the maximal global systolic contraction amplitude.

In the study of Søgaard et al.,[22] patients with idiopathic dilated cardiomyopathy had delayed longitudinal contraction in the lateral and posterior walls of the left ventricle. In contrast, delayed longitudinal contraction was more frequent in the septum and inferior walls in patients with ischemic cardiomyopathy. Preactivation of the left ventricular lead was helpful in 9 patients, and preactivation of the right ventricular lead was superior in the other 11 patients. Left ventricular preactivation tended to be more beneficial in patients with delayed lateral wall contraction (i.e., patients with dilated cardiomyopathy). The degree of preactivation was unexpectedly modest at about 20 milliseconds. It is important to note that the actual area of mechanical asynchrony is not reflected by the left bundle branch block pattern alone but is specific based on the nature of the cardiomyopathy and location of ischemia and infarction. Søgaard et al.[22] also reported significant improvement in the 6-minute hall walk test; the walking distance doubled. This improvement was greater than that reported previously.[8,23,24]

Pitzalis et al.[25] studied mono- and two-dimensional echocardiographic variables in 20 patients with cardiomyopathy. As a group, cardiac resynchronization improved ventricular volumes significantly. However, "responders" were distinguished from "nonresponders" by having a longer interval between contraction of the septum and the posterior wall. The accuracy of septal-to-posterior wall motion delay was greater than that of QRS duration in predicting benefit. It is recognized that chamber enlargement in patients with chronic heart failure is associated with asynchrony between the right and left ventricular walls and between the septum and free wall of the left ventricle. Furthermore, it has been hypothesized that this delayed contraction of the left ventricular free wall contributes to negative remodeling. The clinical benefit to resynchronization therapy, however, is heterogeneous even in patients with demonstrated intraventricular asynchrony. Pitzalis et al.[25] used simple mono-dimensional and two-dimensional echocardiographic recordings to calculate left ventricular end-diastolic and end-systolic volumes. Responders were identified if the left ventricular end-systolic volume index decreased by 15%. Intraventricular asynchrony was evaluated on the basis of left ventricular electromechanical delay, that is, the time from the onset of the QRS complex to aortic ejection. The delay from the septum and left posterior wall was calculated as the shortest interval between maximal posterior displacement of the septum and maximal displacement of the left posterior wall, using a mono-dimensional short-axis view at the level of the papillary muscle.[25]

It should be noted that patients with truly end-stage cardiomyopathy and very large left ventricular volumes are unlikely to benefit from resynchronization,[26] because there is global severe hypokinesia and very little difference between contractility of the septal and free wall regions. It is important to note that in the study by Pitzalis et al.,[25] the baseline PQ interval was by itself of very high predictive value in recognizing responders. Multivariate analysis was not possible in this study, but this may emphasize the value of restoring left atrial and left ventricular synchrony.

Acute hemodynamic data obtained at cardiac catheterization initially showed the benefits of resynchronization therapy on ventricular performance. Noninvasive techniques have been studied; however, the best technique for use long-term and during exercise is not known.[27,28] Radioisotope techniques have low temporal and spatial resolution, making them relatively unsuitable for quantifying the degree of regional left ventricular synchrony.[27,28] Søgaard et al.[22] have used Doppler tissue imaging and three-dimensional echocardiography to quantify regional and global left ventricular function and volumes.[29-31] Tissue tracking and strain rate analysis derived from tissue Doppler imaging can be used to assess intramyocardial asynchrony and have been studied in predicting which patients will have a response to cardiac resynchronization therapy. Tissue tracking visualizes the amplitude of the longitudinal motion in each myocardial section during systole. Strain rate analysis is used to determine whether this motion is active contraction or passive. Both tissue tracking and strain rate analysis have been shown to be useful for evaluating regional myocardial pathophysiology before and after cardiac resynchronization.

Søgaard et al.[22] studied the immediate and long-term benefits of both tissue Doppler imaging and three-dimensional echocardiography after cardiac resynchronization. Twenty-five patients with heart failure and left bundle branch block who underwent biventricular pacemaker implantation were studied with three-dimensional echocardiography and tissue Doppler imaging. Of 20 patients who were alive at the end of 1 year, left ventricular end-diastolic and end-systolic volumes and ventricular function had all improved. Tissue tracking showed that all regional myocardial segments had improved longitudinal systolic shortening. The extent of the left ventricular base that displayed delayed longitudinal contraction (contraction after aortic ejection) as detected with tissue Doppler imaging predicted long-term efficacy of cardiac resynchronization therapy. Of note in this study, the QRS duration did not predict resynchronization efficacy.[22,24]

Yu et al.[32] studied the acute and long-term mechanisms of resynchronization on ventricular modeling using tissue Doppler imaging. With tissue Doppler imaging, the time and peak velocity of contraction of the various ventricular regions were measured. The interventricular variation to peak contraction decreased with resynchronization therapy. This effect was not only immediate but persisted at 1 month after implantation.

Other End Points for Optimization

Although both AV optimization and VV optimization have primarily targeted improvements in mechanical function and, in some instances, its translation to effort tolerance,[24] other end points need to be considered.

Mitral Regurgitation

The extent of mitral regurgitation has been shown to decrease with left ventricular stimulation. It does not follow, however, that the ideal lead location, AV interval, and VV interval for improving cardiac output or ventricular contractility will be the same as those that minimize mitral regurgitation the most.

Arrhythmogenesis

Arrhythmogenesis is known to be enhanced with certain pacing sites and patterns of ventricular activation that cause a widened dispersion in electrical activation. Similarly, certain sites of ventricular activation may be arrhythmogenic compared with other sites. Perhaps the reverse may occur, that is, certain sites of activation can suppress arrhythmogenesis. It does not follow that the optimal sites for pacing and stimulation intervals for ventricular mechanical function will be the same as those that suppress (or at least do not promote) arrhythmogenicity.

Left Atrial Pacing

It is necessary to consider the potential benefit of left atrial pacing to control more directly left atrial-to-left ventricular delay in activation as an adjunct to the benefits observed with ventricular resynchronization alone.

QT Interval

The QT interval can be used as a marker for ideal ventricular output. Ishikawa et al.[33] have shown a correlation between the QT interval and cardiac output and the effect of these measures by varying the paced AV intervals. At optimal AV intervals, an increase is noted in both cardiac output and QT interval.

Diastolic Function

Diastolic function is a complex sequence of events that reflects the relaxing myocardium and diastole. Various factors, including true relaxation, pericardial restraint, atrial contraction, and chamber stiffness, determine the ability of the heart to relax and fill with blood in diastole. Diastolic dysfunction, which is an abnormality of at least one of these factors, occurs frequently in patients with congestive heart failure and cardiomyopathy. Little is known about optimization of biventricular systems in relation to diastolic function. The variables that produce ideal systolic function may be equivocal or perhaps even detrimental to diastolic function. Both AV optimization and VV timing optimization have a role in diastolic function. Optimizing the ventricular lead position and VV timing may indirectly improve relaxation by decreasing negative remodeling and improving myocardial energetics. AV optimization, however, affects diastolic filling by improving the timing of atrial contribution in diastole. Few studies have specifically examined the optimization of diastolic function.[10,24] Tissue tracking and strain rate imaging, both likely to be used increasingly in the future for optimizing systolic function, also provide data about diastolic function.

Optimization of Sensing

Classic biventricular pacing uses the tip electrodes for simultaneous cathodal stimulation of the two ventricles, with the proximal right ventricular ring electrode serving as the common anode. This should be distinguished from split bipolar stimulation that uses the left ventricle as a cathode and the right ventricular tip as the anode. This dual cathodal arrangement should permit a lower biventricular pacing threshold.[34,35] Initial biventricular devices sensed simultaneously from both ventricles, that is, either from the left ventricle to the right ventricular tip or from the combined left and right ventricles to the right ventricular ring. This system may cause double sensing of the QRS complex as well as far-field sensing of the P wave and T wave. This is of concern in biventricular implantable cardioverter-defibrillators because of inappropriate shocks.[36] Temporal separation of the local right ventricular and left ventricular electrograms may cause double counting of the sensed spontaneous conducted ventricular beat when the left ventricular electrogram extends beyond the short blanking period initiated by detection of the right ventricular electrogram. Double counting of the QRS complex occurs in these first-generation systems when pacing is inhibited because of either loss of tracking or tachyarrhythmias. In particularly difficult cases, changing the system or disconnecting the right ventricular lead and pacing of a stable left ventricular lead may be required.

The coronary veins themselves may have electrical activity resulting from their occasionally thick muscular sleeves.[7,37] Far-field sensing of atrial activity either from this coronary sinus source or the neighboring left atrium may inhibit biventricular pacing and induce the emergence of spontaneous AV conduction. This can result in double or triple (atrial and both ventricular signals) counting and the delivery of inappropriate shocks.

Dynamic Optimization

Perhaps most important is dynamic optimization of all the above-mentioned methods of optimizing biventricular system function. That is, whereas a particular lead position VV, VV interval, and AV interval are ideal in the baseline supine state, they may be quite different in a patient who is exercising. In fact, the slope at which these individual variables change with exercise may be different from one another. Thus, individual dynamic optimization of these variables may be required.[38] The existing difficulty of finding a single electrical or electrophysiologic variable that best parallels patient outcomes and can be measured in an ongoing fashion when drugs and patient comorbidity supervene is unsolved. Until such a variable is found, it is arduous to design dynamic algorithms.

Summary

Biventricular device optimization is an important challenge in the care of patients with heart failure. Although many hypotheses have been put forth and some tested in limited fashion, the search continues for the elusive reproducible, easy to measure parameter that parallels patient performance. ECG variables are simple and theoretically elegant in aiding optimization. However, they completely disregard the variable electromechanical delay that occurs from site to site in patients with cardiomyopathy. In comparison, echocardiographic variables have important practical as well as theoretical technical limitations.

References

1. Abraham WT, Fisher WG, Smith AL, Delurgio DB, Leon AR, Lohe H, et al, for the MIRACLE Study Group. Cardiac resynchronization in chronic heart failure. N Engl J Med 2002;346:1845-53.
2. Ansalone G, Trambaiolo P, Giorda GP, Giannantoni P, Ricci R, Santini M. Multisite stimulation in refractory heart failure. G Ital Cardiol 1999;29:451-9.
3. Bradley DJ, Bradley EA, Baughman KL, Berger RD, Calkins H, Goodman SN, et al. Cardiac resynchronization and death from progressive heart failure: a meta-analysis of randomized controlled trials. JAMA 2003;289:730-40.
4. Kass DA, Chen CH, Curry C, Talbot M, Berger R, Fetics B, et al. Improved left ventricular mechanics from acute VDD pacing in patients with dilated cardiomyopathy and ventricular conduction delay. Circulation 1999;99:1567-73.
5. Auricchio A, Stellbrink C, Block M, Sack S, Vogt J, Bakker P, et al, for the Pacing Therapies for Congestive Heart Failure Study Group and the Guidant Congestive Heart Failure Research Group. Effect of pacing chamber and atrioventricular delay on acute systolic function of paced patients with congestive heart failure. Circulation 1999;99:2993-3001.
6. Nishimura RA, Hayes DL, Holmes DR Jr, Tajik AJ. Mechanism of hemodynamic improvement by dual-chamber pacing for severe left ventricular dysfunction: an acute Doppler and catheterization hemodynamic study. J Am Coll Cardiol 1995;25:281-8.
7. Asirvatham S, Packer DL. Longitudinal disassociation of atrial and coronary sinus conduction in man [abstract]. Circulation 2000;102 Suppl 2:II-441.

8. Cazeau S, Leclercq C, Lavergne T, Walker S, Varma C, Linde C, et al, for the Multisite Stimulation in Cardiomyopathies (MUSTIC) Study Investigators. Effects of multisite biventricular pacing in patients with heart failure and intraventricular conduction delay. N Engl J Med 2001;344:873-80.

9. Leclercq C, Cazeau S, Le Breton H, Ritter P, Mabo P, Gras D, et al. Acute hemodynamic effects of biventricular DDD pacing in patients with end-stage heart failure. J Am Coll Cardiol 1998;32:1825-31.

10. Kass DA. Pathophysiology of physiologic cardiac pacing: advantages of leaving well enough alone. JAMA 2002;288;3159-61.

11. Butter C, Auricchio A, Stellbrink C, Fleck E, Ding J, Yu Y, et al, Pacing Therapy for Chronic Heart Failure II (PATH-CHF-II) Study Group. Effect of resynchronization therapy stimulation site on the systolic function of heart failure patients. Circulation 2001;104:3026-9.

12. Ritter P, Padeletti L, Gillio-Meina L, Gaggini G. Determination of the optimal atrioventricular delay in DDD pacing: comparison between echo and peak endocardial acceleration measurements. Europace 1999;1:126-30.

13. Ishikawa T, Kashiwagi M, Usui T, Ochiai H, Ohyama Y, Nakamaru M, et al. Atrioventricular delay and diastolic mitral regurgitation in patient with DDD pacemaker implantation, and cardiac function [Japanese]. Kokyu To Junkan 1990;38:869-74.

14. Ishikawa T, Sumita S, Kimura K, Kuji N, Nakayama R, Nagura T, et al. Critical PQ interval for the appearance of diastolic mitral regurgitation and optimal PQ interval in patients implanted with DDD pacemakers. Pacing Clin Electrophysiol 1994;17:1989-94.

15. Ishikawa T, Kimura K, Miyazaki N, Tochikudo O, Usui T, Kashiwagi M, et al. Diastolic mitral regurgitation in patients with first-degree atrioventricular block. Pacing Clin Electrophysiol 1992;15:1927-31.

16. Tse HF, Yu C, Lee KL, Yu CM, Tsang V, Leung SK, et al. Initial clinical experience with a new self-retaining left ventricular lead for permanent left ventricular pacing. Pacing Clin Electrophysiol 2000;23:1738-40.

17. Ishikawa T, Kimura K, Yoshimura H, Kobayashi K, Usui T, Kashiwagi M, et al. Acute changes in left atrial and left ventricular diameters after physiological pacing. Pacing Clin Electrophysiol 1996;19:143-9.

18. Ricci R, Pignalberi C, Ansalone G, Jannone E, Vaccaro MV, Denaro A, et al. Early and late QRS morphology and width in biventricular pacing: relationship to lead site and electrical remodeling. J Interv Card Electrophysiol 2002;6:279-85.

19. Ansalone G, Giannantoni P, Ricci R, Trambaiolo P, Fedele F, Santini M. Doppler myocardial imaging to evaluate the effectiveness of pacing sites in patients receiving biventricular pacing. J Am Coll Cardiol 2002;39:489-99.

20. Brodin LA, van der Linden J, Olstad B. Echocardiographic functional images based on tissue velocity information. Herz 1998;23:491-8.

21. Wilkenshoff UM, Sovany A, Wigstrom L, Olstad B, Lindstrom L, Engvall J, et al. Regional mean systolic myocardial velocity estimation by real-time color Doppler myocardial imaging: a new technique for quantifying regional systolic function. J Am Soc Echocardiogr 1998;11:683-92.

22. Søgaard P, Kim WY, Jensen HK, Martenson P, Pedersen AK, Kristensen BO, et al. Impact of acute biventricular pacing on left ventricular performance and volumes in patients with severe heart failure: a tissue Doppler and three-dimensional echocardiographic study. Cardiology 2001;95:173-82.

23. Søgaard P, Egeblad H, Kim WY, Jensen HK, Pedersen AK, Kristensen BO, et al. Tissue Doppler imaging predicts improved systolic performance and reversed left ventricular

remodeling during long-term cardiac resynchronization therapy. J Am Coll Cardiol 2002;40:723-30.

24. Søgaard P, Egeblad H, Pedersen AK, Kim WY, Kristensen BO, Hansen PS, et al. Sequential versus simultaneous biventricular resynchronization for severe heart failure: evaluation by tissue Doppler imaging. Circulation 2002;106:2078-84.

25. Pitzalis MV, Iacoviello M, Romito R, Massari F, Rizzon B, Luzzi G, et al. Cardiac resynchronization therapy tailored by echocardiographic evaluation of ventricular asynchrony. J Am Coll Cardiol 2002;40:1615-22.

26. Stellbrink C, Breithardt OA, Franke A, Sack S, Bakker P, Auricchio A, et al, PATH-CHF Investigators and CPI Guidant Congestive Heart Failure Research Group. Impact of cardiac resynchronization therapy using hemodynamically optimized pacing on left ventricular remodeling in patients with congestive heart failure and ventricular conduction disturbances. J Am Coll Cardiol 2001;38:1957-65.

27. Le Rest C, Couturier O, Turzo A, Guillo P, Bizais Y, Etienne Y, et al. Use of left ventricular pacing in heart failure: evaluation by gated blood pool imaging. J Nucl Cardiol 1999;6:651-6.

28. Kerwin WF, Botvinick EH, O'Connell JW, Merrick SH, DeMarco T, Chatterjee K, et al. Ventricular contraction abnormalities in dilated cardiomyopathy: effect of biventricular pacing to correct interventricular dyssynchrony. J Am Coll Cardiol 2000;35:1221-7.

29. Kim WY, Søgaard P, Kristensen BO, Egeblad H. Measurement of left ventricular volumes by 3-dimensional echocardiography with tissue harmonic imaging: a comparison with magnetic resonance imaging. J Am Soc Echocardiogr 2001;14:169-79.

30. Hatle L, Sutherland GR. Regional myocardial function: a new approach. Eur Heart J 2000;21:1337-57.

31. Brodin L-A, Gabella M, van der Linden J, Madler C, Olstad B. Simultaneous display of tissue velocity and strain: a fast option in evaluation of myocardial function [abstract]. J Am Coll Cardiol 2001;37 Suppl A:410A.

32. Yu CM, Chau E, Sanderson JE, Fan K, Tang MO, Fung WH, et al. Tissue Doppler echocardiographic evidence of reverse remodeling and improved synchronicity by simultaneously delaying regional contraction after biventricular pacing therapy in heart failure. Circulation 2002;105:438-45.

33. Ishikawa T, Sugano T, Sumita S, Kimura K, Kikuchi M, Kosuge M, et al. Relationship between atrioventricular delay, QT interval and cardiac function in patients with implanted DDD pacemakers. Europace 1999;1:192-6.

34. Barold SS, Byrd CL. Cross-ventricular endless loop tachycardia during biventricular pacing. Pacing Clin Electrophysiol 2001;24:1821-3.

35. Barold SS, Levine PA. Significance of stimulation impedance in biventricular pacing. J Interv Card Electrophysiol 2002;6:67-70.

36. Schreieck J, Zrenner B, Kolb C, Ndrepepa G, Schmitt C. Inappropriate shock delivery due to ventricular double detection with a biventricular pacing implantable cardioverter defibrillator. Pacing Clin Electrophysiol 2001;24:1154-7.

37. Lipchenca I, Garrigue S, Glikson M, Barold SS, Clementy J. Inhibition of biventricular pacemakers by oversensing or far-field atrial depolarization. Pacing Clin Electrophysiol 2002;25:365-7.

38. Leung SK, Lau CP, Lam CT, Ho S, Tse HF, Yu CM, et al. Automatic optimization of resting and exercise atrioventricular interval using a peak endocardial acceleration sensor: validation with Doppler echocardiography and direct cardiac output measurements. Pacing Clin Electrophysiol 2000;23:1762-6.

CHAPTER 6

What Echocardiography May Offer Cardiac Resynchronization Therapy

Theodore P. Abraham, MD

Why include a chapter on the role of echocardiography in cardiac resynchronization therapy (CRT)? As the discipline of CRT evolves, it is clear there are many areas for improvement, including patient selection, device optimization, and follow-up. Clearly, echocardiography has a role both before and after CRT implantation. However, the full potential of echocardiography in this discipline has not been realized. Some of the echocardiographic techniques discussed in this chapter are new and not well validated—they are not the "standard of care" for CRT patients. Subsequent editions of this text and certainly this chapter are likely to be vastly different, and it may be more appropriate to include the information about echocardiography in the sections on patient selection and optimization.

Preimplantation Echocardiography

Preimplantation echocardiography is immensely beneficial in patients being considered for CRT. For several reasons, echocardiography may be the preferred imaging modality to assess patients before CRT (Table 1). Echocardiography helps to establish

---

Table 1. Potential Advantages of Echocardiography in CRT Evaluation

Noninvasive modality
Evaluates remodeling, hemodynamics, and mechanical synchrony
Portable and can be used in the electrophysiology laboratory
Compatible with all electrophysiology devices
Does not obstruct the operator's field during imaging
Echocardiography parameters can be easily applied to clinical situations because
 most clinical trial data were based on echocardiography

CRT, cardiac resynchronization therapy.

the baseline cardiac morphology and hemodynamics, thus allowing subsequent monitoring of cardiac remodeling and hemodynamic changes after CRT. Standard morphologic parameters measured before implantation include left ventricular end-systolic and end-diastolic diameters and volumes and ejection fraction. Doppler studies are used to define diastolic function, severity of mitral regurgitation, and interventricular mechanical delay (the difference in time to onset of flow in the right ventricular outflow tract compared with the left ventricular outflow tract). Septal-to-lateral wall motion delay can also be evaluated using the M-mode of the mid ventricular short-axis view (Fig. 1).[1] This measurement may prove valuable for assessing patients before CRT and for optimizing the implanted device. This is described below.

Echocardiography may have a major role in identifying patients who will respond to CRT. Limited data from small studies indicate that echocardiographic parameters may be more accurate than electrocardiographic (ECG) and clinical parameters. For example, QRS width often does not change after CRT and the evidence is conflicting about whether baseline QRS width predicts who will respond to CRT.[1] Furthermore, results from animal studies suggest that electrical and mechanical synchrony are not related.[2] In one animal study, investigators demonstrated that correction of mechanical asynchrony resulted in notable hemodynamic improvement despite no change in electrical synchrony. Also, reported data suggest that conventional echocardiography may not suffice for the evaluation of patients before or after CRT. In a small study, septal-to-posterior wall motion delay was shown to predict improvement whereas other parameters such as QRS width and interventricular mechanical delay were not predictive.[1] The utility of this simple variable will have to be confirmed in larger and longer term studies. Echocardiographic data derived from current clinical studies were obtained from post hoc comparisons of "responders" versus "nonresponders." Some of the echocardiographic parameters that indicate interventricular and intraventricular dyssynchrony are presented in Table 2 and Figures 2 and 3.[1,3-6] To date, prospective data as to which echocardiographic parameters best predict response are limited.

In addition to M-mode and two-dimensional echocardiographic techniques that are commonly used and understood, several newer echocardiographic applications are emerging that have potential application to CRT, during both patient selection and follow-up. Because of the newness of these techniques and the lack of general familiarity, a brief explanation of the basic techniques is required before their potential CRT applications are discussed.

Tissue Doppler Strain Echocardiography

Tissue Doppler strain echocardiography has been used to assess regional mechanical synchrony.[3,5] Tissue Doppler imaging is an extension of conventional Doppler echocardiography and may provide additional functional information. High-frequency, low-amplitude echoes originating from the blood pool are filtered out and

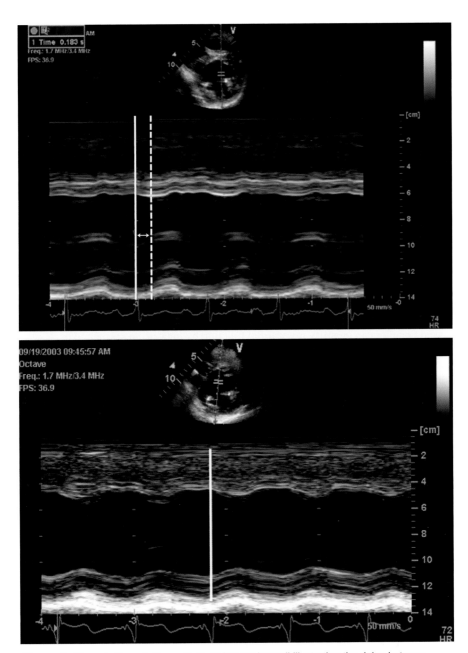

Figure 1. M-mode through the septum and posterior wall illustrating the delay between onset of systolic thickening in the septal (solid white line) versus the posterior wall (dashed white line). In this example, pre-CRT (top) delay was ~180 ms and onset of systolic thickening is almost simultaneous post-CRT (solid white line) (bottom).

Table 2. Echocardiographic Parameters of Dyssynchrony

Interventricular dyssynchrony
  Difference in time to onset of flow in right versus left ventricular outflow
    tract—mean delay was ~45 ms in CRT responders
Intraventricular dyssynchrony
  Septal-to-lateral wall motion delay by M-mode echocardiography—mean
    delay in responders pre-CRT was 192 ms and decreased to 14 ms post-CRT;
    proposed cutoff for responders was >130 ms
  Standard deviation of time to peak systolic tissue velocity in basal and mid
    segments—mean delay was 37 ms pre-CRT and decreased to 29 ms post-
    CRT
  Percent of basal segments demonstrating delayed longitudinal contraction on
    tissue tracking was >20 in CRT responders

CRT, cardiac resynchronization therapy.

myocardial tissue velocity is expressed as a color or spectral display (Fig. 4).[7-9] Tissue Doppler can quantify myocardial function by measuring segmental peak systolic and diastolic tissue velocities. However, because tissue Doppler measures the velocity at a single point in the myocardium, it is influenced adversely by cardiac translational motion and does not efficiently discriminate between actively contracting and tethered myocardium.[10] Also, in the longitudinal plane, the apex is mostly stationary and the maximum motion occurs at the base. Thus, tissue velocities are usually highest at the base and lowest or absent at the apex (Fig. 5). There is a gradient in tissue velocities proceeding from the base to the apex. The gradient is exploited to calculate strain rate. However, because of this gradient, tissue velocities vary from the base to the apex, which makes it challenging to assign cutoff points for peak tissue velocities in most segments except the basal ones.

Tissue Displacement

Tissue velocities can be integrated to yield tissue displacement. Therefore, if tissue velocity is the velocity of tissue motion at a particular point in the myocardium, then tissue displacement is the total distance that particular point travels. Tissue displacement of various segments of the myocardium can be color-coded and represented on the monitor as an easily read color map (Fig. 6). This technique is called "tissue tracking" by one vendor. In the tissue-tracking mode, the end frame is set at end-systole. The program colors each segment depending on the distance that particular segment traveled between the time points identified by the operator. The time points are usually set to capture all systolic motion; thus, the

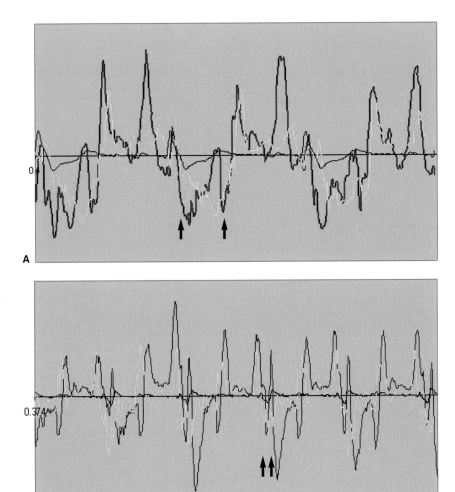

Figure 2. Strain rate profiles of septal (blue) and lateral (yellow) basal segments (arrows, peak systolic strain rate). Note the reduction in time delay between septal and lateral walls post-CRT (B) compared with pre-CRT (A). Black line, ECG.

first marker is set to just after the R wave of the ECG and the end marker is set to peak systole or at the time of aortic valve closure. Tissue tracking has been used to track segments that have delayed contraction. If an electronic time marker (on the machine) is set after aortic valve closure (end of global systole), the segments showing tissue displacement after that time point have delayed contraction patterns, which will be displayed as colored segments on tissue tracking. The observer can note the number of basal segments that are still colored after aortic

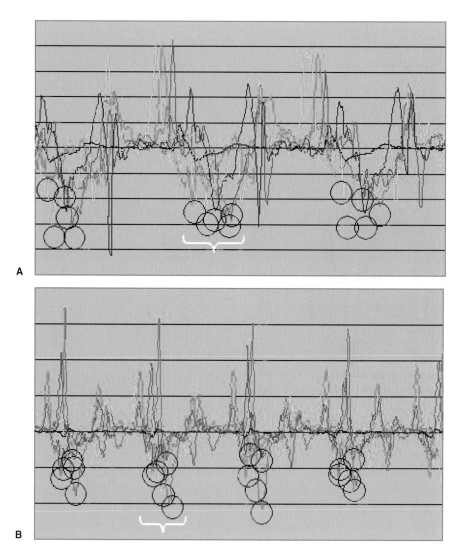

Figure 3. A, Example of measurement of time to peak systolic strain rate in all basal segments from the apical views only (circles, peak systolic strain rate) measured pre-CRT. White braces, the time spread between the minimum and maximum delay. B, The spread between the minimum and maximum time intervals is substantially reduced post-CRT.

valve closure and determine the percentage of segments that have delayed contraction. Data indicate that CRT responders usually have delayed contraction in more than 20% of the basal segments. This delayed contraction pattern can be confirmed by placing a region of interest in the "delayed segment" and confirming the delay in peak systole by tissue velocity or strain rate.[3,11]

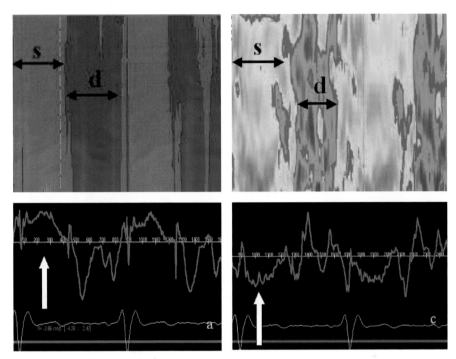

Figure 4. Upper left, Tissue Doppler color and, lower left, velocity profiles. Upper right, Strain rate color and, lower right, profile. See text for details. s, systole; d, diastole. White arrow, peak systolic tissue velocity or strain rate.

Tissue Synchronization Imaging

Tissue synchronization imaging (TSI) is an attempt to help clinicians identify in a semiautomated manner segments that have delayed contraction. In this mode, the operator sets a cutoff time point on the machine. The machine then looks for the time to peak systolic tissue velocity and colors all segments that achieve their peak before the time cutoff different from those that peak after the time point (Fig. 7). Because the tissue velocity signal is usually robust and clear, automated identification of the peak systolic tissue velocity is relatively easy. Time points can be set arbitrarily or set to aortic valve closure.

Strain Rate Imaging

The calculation of local strain rates (also called "velocity gradients," depending on the technique) can be made from tissue Doppler data. Strain rate measures the mechanical behavior of two points within the myocardium by determining the difference between tissue velocities at those two points.[12-15] Thus, when the

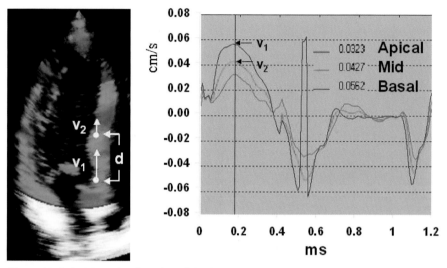

Figure 5. Left, A four-chamber view of the heart with tissue velocities measured at two points on the myocardium (V₁ and V₂). The difference in these two velocities normalized for the distance, d, between the two points is strain rate. Right, Tissue velocity traces taken from apical, mid, and basal segments illustrating the velocity gradient (decremental velocity from base to apex).

myocardium is contracting, it shortens in the longitudinal axis and the two points come closer to each other. The rate at which these two points converge in systole is "strain rate" and the distance they travel toward each other is "strain." In physical terms, strain is length change and strain rate is the rate of length change. Strain is defined as the change in length normalized to the initial length of the myocardium

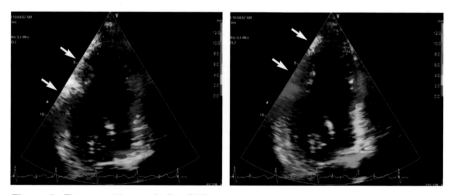

Figure 6. Tissue tracking. Left, Pre-CRT images demonstrate delayed tissue motion (no color) in the lateral apical region (arrows) compared to the septum. Right, This region shows normal tissue motion post-CRT.

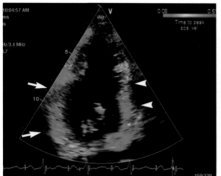 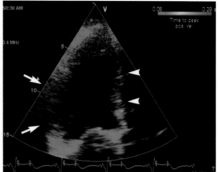

Figure 7. Left, Tissue resynchronization imaging (TSI) demonstrates that the basal and mid-lateral wall segments (arrows) have a delayed time to peak systolic tissue velocity compared with the septal wall, pre-CRT. In this example, the TSI cutoff pre-CRT was set at 53 ms, which indicates that all segments achieving peak systolic tissue motion in <53 ms were displayed in gray scale (arrowheads) and those achieving peak systolic motion >53 ms were displayed in yellow-green-red (arrows). Right, Post-CRT, the lateral segments move concordant with the septal segments as indicated by both lateral (arrows) and septal (arrowheads) walls displayed in gray scale. The post-CRT TSI cutoff was set at 27 ms, which means all segments achieving peak systolic tissue motion in <27 ms were displayed in gray scale.

and is therefore expressed as a percentage (change in length as a percentage of original length). Because the length at peak systole is shorter than the original length, strain (and strain rate) has a negative polarity when measured in the longitudinal length.[16] The opposite occurs in the short-axis (radial) plane when the myocardium thickens during systole, and in this plane, systolic strain rate and strain have positive polarity. The polarity of the diastolic waves is the opposite of that of the systolic wave and is positive in the longitudinal direction and negative in the short-axis (radial) direction. Strain rate measures the activity of two points within the myocardium; therefore, it is less susceptible to cardiac translation and tethering artifacts.

Application of Newer Echocardiographic Techniques to CRT

Tissue Doppler–based assessment of regional (intraventricular) synchrony has been shown to be useful.[3-5,11] There appears to be no marked change in regional contractile function as reflected by the absence of a notable increase in regional strain rate and strain with CRT.[17] However, the improvement in global function is probably related more to a coordinated systolic motion of individual myocardial segments. The standard deviation of the time to peak systolic tissue velocity has been shown to decrease in responders compared with nonresponders (Fig. 3).[4] Similarly, delayed longitudinal segmental contractions as demonstrated by tissue tracking (tissue displacement) or strain rate may be useful. The presence of delayed longitudinal contraction in more than 20% of the basal segments on all three apical views has been shown to be predictive of clinical improvement.[3] Tissue Doppler strain echocardiography can also be used to measure septal-to-lateral wall motion delay to mimic the previously described M-mode measurement (Fig. 2).

Regardless of the technique or parameter, these data have limitations in helping to identify echocardiographic predictors of response to CRT. Most of the studies have involved a small number of patients and have been primarily retrospective in design. Because intraventricular delays were the inclusion criteria for CRT, the finding that intraventricular delays predict clinical response may have inherent bias. However, recent advances in echocardiographic technology may allow easier clinical application of novel, quantitative imaging strategies, which may also identify CRT responders.

Role of Echocardiography at the Time of Implantation

According to preliminary evidence, echocardiography can be used at the time of implantation to assess mechanical synchrony and to appropriately guide the operator to implant the left ventricular lead at the optimal site. It is known that certain left ventricular pacing sites are not associated with clinical improvement.[18] Some investigators have proposed placing the left ventricular lead in the segments (wall) with the longest delay in systolic contraction, as indicated by tissue Doppler strain imaging. Ideally, this should result in the most coordinated left ventricular contraction. If tissue Doppler strain studies indicate suboptimal coordination, the pacing could be altered to find the most suitable location for the left ventricular lead. Although no data have been published on the role of echocardiography at implantation, ongoing clinical trials seek to address this issue.

Postimplantation Use of Echocardiography for Follow-up and Optimization

As discussed in the chapter on CRT optimization, echocardiography has been used extensively for optimization of the atrioventricular (AV) interval and more recently for ventricle-to-ventricle (VV) optimization. Currently, AV interval optimization is being done with the Ritter technique as well as with an iterative technique, that is, gradually incrementing or decrementing the programmed AV interval in an effort to fine-tune hemodynamics by assessing mitral inflow patterns and optimizing the separation of the e and a waves. Other variations of echocardiographic optimization have been described.[19,20] The left ventricular outflow tract time velocity integral has been used to optimize VV timing. This technique has several limitations. The time velocity integral is highly load dependent and there is considerable beat-to-beat variability. The time velocity integral signal depends on the

Doppler angle, and if the peak velocity is not obtained, the time velocity integral will be erroneous. There is interest in developing new parameters, possibly tissue Doppler strain–based, to better assess the efficacy of VV timing. These new parameters need to be validated clinically.

During follow-up, echocardiography allows assessment of myocardial remodeling. Most clinical CRT studies have demonstrated positive remodeling, that is, a decrease in left ventricular end-systolic and end-diastolic diameters and volumes.[18,21-23] Although some studies have shown an increase in left ventricular ejection fraction, the increase has been modest in long-term studies. Echocardiography has also demonstrated a decrease in the severity of mitral regurgitation.[24] Improvement in mitral regurgitation may contribute to improvement in symptoms and positive remodeling.

Future Directions

Echocardiography may contribute in several ways to optimizing delivery of CRT therapy. Some potential issues that may be addressed using conventional or novel echocardiographic techniques include the following:

- To determine if left ventricular outflow tract time velocity integral is the best parameter to ascertain the optimal VV timing
- To track changes in diastolic filling with CRT
- To identify noninvasive predictors of CRT response
- To help guide location of left ventricular lead placement and to test whether guided left ventricular lead placement provides superior clinical benefits to "blind" left ventricular lead placement
- To determine the role of regional infarction and myocardial viability on long-term clinical outcomes and whether echocardiography can help address these issues

References

1. Pitzalis MV, Iacoviello M, Romito R, Massari F, Rizzon B, Luzzi G, et al. Cardiac resynchronization therapy tailored by echocardiographic evaluation of ventricular asynchrony. J Am Coll Cardiol 2002;40:1615-22.

2. Leclercq C, Faris O, Tunin R, Johnson J, Kato R, Evans F, et al. Systolic improvement and mechanical resynchronization does not require electrical synchrony in the dilated failing heart with left bundle-branch block. Circulation 2002;106:1760-3.

3. Søgaard P, Egeblad H, Kim WY, Jensen HK, Pedersen AK, Kristensen BO, et al. Tissue Doppler imaging predicts improved systolic performance and reversed left ventricular remodeling during long-term cardiac resynchronization therapy. J Am Coll Cardiol 2002;40:723-30.

4. Yu CM, Chau E, Sanderson JE, Fan K, Tang MO, Fung WH, et al. Tissue Doppler echocardiographic evidence of reverse remodeling and improved synchronicity by simultaneously delaying regional contraction after biventricular pacing therapy in heart failure. Circulation 2002;105:438-45.

5. Yu CM, Fung WH, Lin H, Zhang Q, Sanderson JE, Lau CP. Predictors of left ventricular reverse remodeling after cardiac resynchronization therapy for heart failure secondary to idiopathic dilated or ischemic cardiomyopathy. Am J Cardiol 2003;91:684-8.

6. Yu CM, Lin H, Fung WH, Zhang Q, Kong SL, Sanderson JE. Comparison of acute changes in left ventricular volume, systolic and diastolic functions, and intraventricular synchronicity after biventricular and right ventricular pacing for heart failure. Am Heart J 2003;145:E18.

7. Sutherland GR, Stewart MJ, Groundstroem KW, Moran CM, Fleming A, Guell-Peris FJ, et al. Color Doppler myocardial imaging: a new technique for the assessment of myocardial function. J Am Soc Echocardiogr 1994;7:441-58.

8. Wilkenshoff UM, Sovany A, Wigstrom L, Olstad B, Lindstrom L, Engvall J, et al. Regional mean systolic myocardial velocity estimation by real-time color Doppler myocardial imaging: a new technique for quantifying regional systolic function. J Am Soc Echocardiogr 1998;11:683-92.

9. García-Fernández MA, Zamorano J, Azevedo J. Doppler tissue imaging echocardiography. Madrid: McGraw-Hill; 1998.

10. Abraham TP, Nishimura RA, Holmes DR Jr, Belohlavek M, Seward JB. Strain rate imaging for assessment of regional myocardial function: results from a clinical model of septal ablation. Circulation 2002;105:1403-6.

11. Søgaard P, Egeblad H, Pedersen AK, Kim WY, Kristensen BO, Hansen PS, et al. Sequential versus simultaneous biventricular resynchronization for severe heart failure: evaluation by tissue Doppler imaging. Circulation 2002;106:2078-84.

12. Abraham TP, Laskowski C, Zhan WZ, Belohlavek M, Martin EA, Greenleaf JF, et al. Myocardial contractility by strain echocardiography: comparison with physiological measurements in an in vitro model. Am J Physiol Heart Circ Physiol 2003;285:H2599-604.

13. Edvardsen T, Gerber BL, Bluemke DA, Lima JAC, Smiseth OA. Doppler derived strain in myocardial infarction: validation versus magnetic resonance imaging with tissue tagging (abstract). Circulation 1999;100 Suppl 1:I-776.

14. Heimdal A, Stoylen A, Torp H, Skjaerpe T. Real-time strain rate imaging of the left ventricle by ultrasound. J Am Soc Echocardiogr 1998;11:1013-9.

15. Urheim S, Edvardsen T, Torp H, Angelsen B, Smiseth OA. Myocardial strain by Doppler echocardiography: validation of a new method to quantify regional myocardial function. Circulation 2000;102:1158-64.

16. Abraham TP, Nishimura RA. Myocardial strain: can we finally measure contractility? J Am Coll Cardiol 2001;37:731-4.
17. Popovic ZB, Grimm RA, Perlic G, Chinchoy E, Geraci M, Sun JP, et al. Noninvasive assessment of cardiac resynchronization therapy for congestive heart failure using myocardial strain and left ventricular peak power as parameters of myocardial synchrony and function. J Cardiovasc Electrophysiol 2002;13:1203-8.
18. Stellbrink C, Breithardt OA, Franke A, Sack S, Bakker P, Auricchio A, et al., the PATH-CHF Investigators and the CPI Guidant Congestive Heart Failure Research Group. Impact of cardiac resynchronization therapy using hemodynamically optimized pacing on left ventricular remodeling in patients with congestive heart failure and ventricular conduction disturbances. J Am Coll Cardiol 2001;38:1957-65.
19. Ishikawa T, Sumita S, Kimura K, Kikuchi M, Kosuge M, Kuji N, et al. Prediction of optimal atrioventricular delay in patients with implanted DDD pacemakers. Pacing Clin Electrophysiol 1999;22:1365-71.
20. Ishikawa T, Sumita S, Kimura K, Kikuchi M, Matsushita K, Ohkusu Y, et al. Optimization of atrioventricular delay and follow-up in a patient with congestive heart failure and with bi-ventricular pacing. Jpn Heart J 2001;42:781-7.
21. Abraham WT, Fisher WG, Smith AL, Delurgio DB, Leon AR, Loh E, et al., for the MIRACLE Study Group. Cardiac resynchronization in chronic heart failure. N Engl J Med 2002;346:1845-53.
22. Cazeau S, Leclercq C, Lavergne T, Walker S, Varma C, Linde C, et al., for the Multisite Stimulation in Cardiomyopathies (MUSTIC) Study Investigators. Effects of multisite biventricular pacing in patients with heart failure and intraventricular conduction delay. N Engl J Med 2001;344:873-80.
23. Thackray S, Coletta A, Jones P, Dunn A, Clark AL, Cleland JG. Clinical trials update: Highlights of the Scientific Sessions of Heart Failure 2001, a meeting of the Working Group on Heart Failure of the European Society of Cardiology. CONTAK-CD, CHRISTMAS, OPTIME-CHF. Eur J Heart Fail 2001;3:491-4.
24. Breithardt OA, Sinha AM, Schwammenthal E, Bidaoui N, Markus KU, Franke A, et al. Acute effects of cardiac resynchronization therapy on functional mitral regurgitation in advanced systolic heart failure [published erratum appears in J Am Coll Cardiol 2003;41:1852]. J Am Coll Cardiol 2003;41:765-70.

CHAPTER 7

Implantable Defibrillators and Combined ICD-Resynchronization Therapy in Patients With Heart Failure

Paul J. Wang, MD
David L. Hayes, MD

Introduction

Implantable cardioverter-defibrillators (ICDs) have become the central therapy for patients with sustained ventricular arrhythmias. The evolution of ICD therapy has been amazingly rapid; major events in the evolution of ICDs are shown in Figure 1.

Major technologic advances have simplified ICD implantation techniques and have led to widespread application of this therapy.[1] Careful randomized studies have demonstrated increased survival with ICD therapy for both patients with sustained ventricular arrhythmias (secondary prevention) and those at risk for having ventricular arrhythmias (primary prevention). Despite these advances, it is generally accepted that ICD therapy has been offered to only a small fraction of patients who qualify (Fig. 2).

Evidence of improved quality of life for patients with heart failure, left ventricular dysfunction, and widened QRS is rapidly expanding the indications for resynchronization therapy. For many of these patients who are also at risk for having life-threatening ventricular arrhythmias, ICD therapy with resynchronization therapy may be the best option.

Clinical Trials of ICDs for Primary and Secondary Prevention

ICDs for Secondary Prevention

Since the advent of ICD therapy in 1980, this discipline has "grown up" in the age of evidence-based medicine. Clinical trials that have assessed ICD therapy have followed a progression, with overlap, from secondary prevention to primary

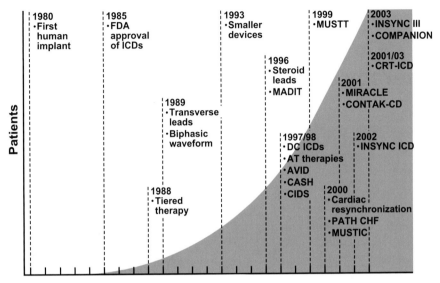

Figure 1. Evolution of ICD therapy. FDA, U.S. Food and Drug Administration. (Modified from Seidl K, Senges J. Worldwide utilization of implantable cardioverter/defibrillators now and in the future. Cardiac Electrophysiol Rev 2003;7:5-13. By permission of Kluwer Academic Publishers.)

prevention to ICD therapies for specific subsets of patients and, finally, to ICD therapy in combination with cardiac resynchronization (Fig. 3).

ICDs have been shown to be effective in preventing sudden cardiac death, with sudden death rates of only 1%. Retrospective studies demonstrated that ICDs were superior to amiodarone therapy. However, because they were retrospective, these studies could not demonstrate that ICDs improve total survival. Several randomized clinical trials demonstrated the effectiveness of ICDs in improving total survival in comparison with drug therapy. Although these are the most definitive trials for secondary prevention, only a small number of patients had severe heart failure. On the basis of these data, it is assumed that ICD therapy provides survival benefit to patients who have heart failure and sustained ventricular arrhythmias.

The Antiarrhythmics versus Implantable Defibrillators (AVID) trial,[2] sponsored by the National Heart, Lung, and Blood Institute, compared ICD therapy with amiodarone or sotalol therapy. Patients with ventricular fibrillation or hemodynamically unstable ventricular tachycardia were eligible. They were randomly assigned to ICD or antiarrhythmic therapy consisting of amiodarone or sotalol. Patients who were not candidates for sotalol were assigned to amiodarone. Patients who were candidates for sotalol initially were randomly assigned to amiodarone or sotalol. In the majority of patients assigned to sotalol therapy, this treatment was not able to suppress the arrhythmia; these patients were given amiodarone. Patients in the ICD

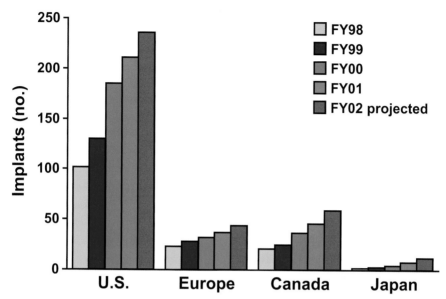

Figure 2. Comparisons of the number of ICD implants in 1998 (FY98) to 2002 (FY02) in the United States, Europe, Canada, and Japan. (Modified from Seidl K, Senges J. Worldwide utilization of implantable cardioverter/defibrillators now and in the future. Cardiac Electrophysiol Rev 2003;7:5-13. By permission of Kluwer Academic Publishers.)

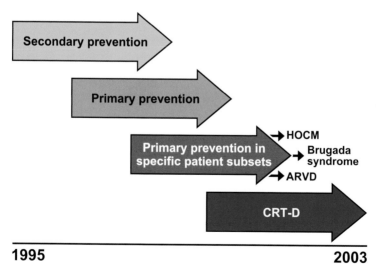

Figure 3. Evolution of ICD randomized clinical trials by type of trial. ARVD, arrhythmogenic right ventricular dysplasia; CRT-D, resynchronization plus ICD therapy; HOCM, hypertrophic obstructive cardiomyopathy.

group had a lower mortality than those in the antiarrhythmic drug group, with decreased death rates at 1, 2, and 3 years. The average unadjusted length of additional life associated with ICD therapy was 2.7 months at 3 years.

Another major prospective ICD trial was the Cardiac Arrest Study Hamburg (CASH) (Germany).[3] Patients were eligible for this study if they had a cardiac arrest not due to a reversible cause. The primary end point was all-cause mortality, but the secondary end point was sudden death. At a mean follow-up of 57±34 months, there was a trend toward improved survival ($P=0.08$) and a significantly greater freedom from sudden death or cardiac arrest ($P=0.005$) in the ICD arm.

The Canadian Implantable Defibrillator Study (CIDS), a secondary prevention trial, examined survival with ICD therapy versus amiodarone therapy.[4] Patients who had ventricular fibrillation or hemodynamically unstable ventricular tachycardia were eligible for the study and were randomly assigned to ICD or amiodarone therapy. There was a trend for improved all-cause mortality and a trend toward freedom from sudden death.

In summary, several randomized trials, including AVID, CASH, and CIDS, provide substantial evidence that ICDs improve survival of patients with sustained ventricular arrhythmias (Table 1, Fig. 4).

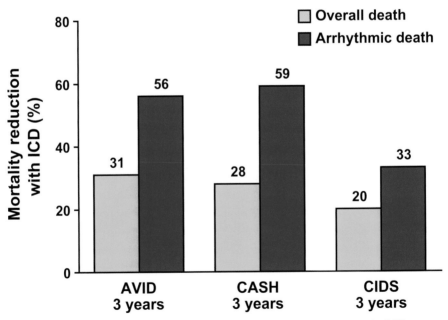

Figure 4. Reduction in mortality with ICD therapy in secondary prevention trials AVID, CASH, and CIDS.

Although a small proportion of patients in these studies have had heart failure, it generally is accepted that patients who have heart failure with sustained ventricular arrhythmias should receive ICD therapy.

ICD Therapy for Primary Prevention of Sudden Cardiac Death and Relevance to Patients With Heart Failure

From the time ICD therapy was approved by the U.S. Food and Drug Administration (FDA) in 1985, the only indication was sustained ventricular arrhythmia. However,

---

Table 1. Comparison of Secondary Prevention Trials

Trial	Inclusion criteria	End point	Study design	Primary results
AVID[2]	VF, sustained VT with syncope, sustained VT with LVEF ≤40% and severe symptoms (near syncope, CHF, angina)	Total mortality	Randomized to ICD or best antiarrhythmic drug (amiodarone or sotalol—EP guided)	Improved survival in ICD group, with average unadjusted length of additional life of 2.7 mo at 3 years
CASH[3]	Cardiac arrest not within 72 h of acute MI, cardiac surgery, electrolyte abnormalities, and a proarrhythmic drug	Primary end point: all-cause mortality. Secondary end points: sudden death & recurrence of cardiac arrest	Randomized to ICD or drug-treatment. In drug arm, 3 antiarrhythmic agents: amiodarone 1,000 mg/day load, then 200-600 mg/day), metoprolol (12.5-25 mg/day increased to maximum 200 mg/day), and propafenone (1:1:1)	Propafenone discontinued in 1992 because of excess mortality. At mean follow-up of 57±34 mo, death rates were 36.4% in ICD and 44.4% in antiarrhythmic arm (1-sided $P=0.081$); crude sudden death 13.0% in ICD and 33.0% in antiarrhythmic arm (1-sided $P=0.005$)

Table 1 (continued)

Trial	Inclusion criteria	End point	Study design	Primary results
CIDS[4]	Documented VF, out-of-hospital cardiac arrest, sustained VT causing syncope, VT >150 bpm causing presyncope or angina; LVEF <35%, unmonitored syncope with inducible VT	All-cause mortality, total & arrhythmic death within 30 days	Randomized to ICD or amiodarone (>1,200 mg/day for ≥10 wk, then ≥300 mg/day	All-cause mortality was 8.3% ICD vs. 10.2% antiarrhythmic drug arm (*P*=0.142) Arrhythmic death was 3.0% ICD vs. 4.5% antiarrhythmic drug arm (*P*=0.094)

bpm, beats/minute; CHF, congestive heart failure; EP, electrophysiologic; LVEF, left ventricular ejection fraction; MI, myocardial infarction; VF, ventricular fibrillation; VT, ventricular tachycardia.

11 years later, in 1996, the FDA approved the first prophylactic use of ICDs. Although numerous studies have examined the likelihood of sudden death for a patient with left ventricular dysfunction, the Multicenter Automatic Defibrillation Implantation Trial (MADIT) I[5] and Multicenter Unsustained Tachycardia Trial (MUSTT)[6] have done the most to promote the use of ICDs for primary prevention of sudden death in patients with coronary artery disease, left ventricular dysfunction, and nonsustained ventricular tachycardia (Table 2, Fig. 5).

Not only are the data unequivocal that ICDs have a major effect on primary prevention of sudden cardiac death, but they also show that the decrease in mortality in the primary prevention trials is equal to or greater than that in the secondary prevention trials described above (compare Figures 4 and 5). However, many of the patients in these studies were not representative of typical patients with heart failure.

In AVID, a post hoc analysis of survival by left ventricular ejection fraction was performed. As demonstrated in Figure 6, the lower the left ventricular ejection fraction the greater the effect ICD had on survival.

Whereas 63% to 67% of patients in MADIT I were listed as having New York Heart Association (NYHA) class II or III heart failure, only 51% to 52% had received treatment for heart failure. The left ventricular ejection fraction was quite low, 25%±7% in the conventional therapy group and 27%±7% in the defibrillator group,

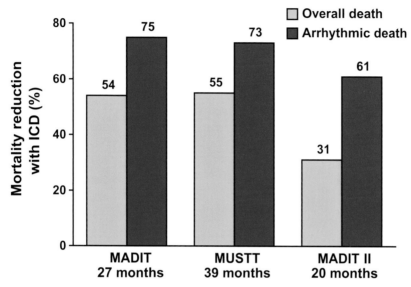

Figure 5. Reduction in mortality with ICD therapy in primary prevention trials MADIT,[1] MUSTT,[16] and MADIT II.[17,18]

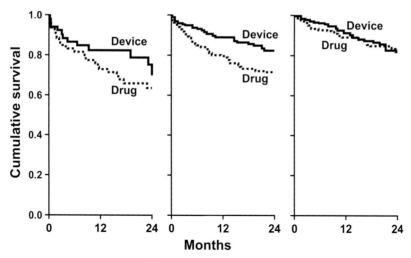

Figure 6. Survival curves from AVID post hoc analyses demonstrating survival by left ventricular ejection fraction. The subset of patients with the lowest left ventricular ejection fraction (<20%, left) had the greatest reduction in mortality. (From Domanski MJ, Sakseena S, Epstein AE, Hallstrom AP, Brodsky MA, Kim S, et al. Relative effectiveness of the implantable cardioverter-defibrillator and antiarrhythmic drugs in patients with varying degrees of left ventricular dysfunction who have survived malignant ventricular arrhythmias. J Am Coll Cardiol 1999;34:1092-95. By permission of the American College of Cardiology.)

but only 20% and 18% of the patients, respectively, had radiographic evidence of pulmonary congestion. Also, the low incidence of left bundle branch block, 8% in the conventional therapy group and 7% in the defibrillator group, suggests that the MADIT I population was not representative of the patients with heart failure currently being treated. Nonetheless, a post hoc analysis again demonstrated that ICD therapy had a greater effect on survival of patients with a lower left ventricular ejection fraction (Fig. 7).

Table 2. Comparison of Primary Prevention Trials

Trial	Inclusion criteria	Primary end point	Study design	Primary results
MADIT[5]	Q-wave MI ≥3 wk; 3-30 beats NSVT; LVEF ≤35%; NYHA I-III; inducible VT not suppressed by procainamide	All-cause mortality	ICD vs. conventional medical therapy	ICDs reduced mortality (hazard ratio for overall mortality, 0.46; 95% CI, 0.26-0.82; $P=0.009$)
CABG-PATCH[7]	CABG, LVEF <36%; abnormal SAECG	All-cause mortality	ICD vs. conventional therapy at time of CABG	No difference in mortality
MUSTT[6]	CAD, LVEF ≤40%, NSVT, inducible VT or VF	Cardiac arrest or arrhythmic death	Antiarrhythmic drug therapy in suppressible patients ICD in non-suppressible patients vs. no therapy	Group with ICDs had 0.24 relative risk of arrhythmic death or cardiac arrest & >50% reduction in total mortality compared with group without ICDs

Table 2 (continued)

Trial	Inclusion criteria	Primary end point	Study design	Primary results
MADIT II[8]	MI >1 mo, LVEF <30%	All-cause mortality	ICD vs. no ICD	ICD group had 14.2% mortality compared with 19.8% for no ICD group at mean follow-up of 20 mo (hazard ratio for risk of death, 0.69; 95% CI, 0.51-0.93; P=0.016)
CAT[9]	Nonischemic CMP diagnosed ≤9 mo, LVEF ≤30%	All-cause mortality	ICD vs. no ICD	No difference in mortality
AMIOVERT[10]	Nonischemic CMP, NSVT, LVEF ≤35%	All-cause mortality, quality of life	Amiodarone vs. ICD	No difference in mortality
SCD-HeFT[11]	NYHA II or III CHF, LVEF ≤35%	All-cause mortality	Placebo vs. amiodarone vs. ICD	In progress
DEFINITE[12]*	Nonischemic CMP, LVEF ≤35%, 3-15–beat NSVT or >10 PVCs/hour	All-cause mortality	CHF medical therapy vs. CHF therapy + ICD	2-y mortality: No ICD, 13.8% ICD, 8.1% RR = 34% Arrhythmia deaths decreased (RR = 74%, P=0.01)
DINAMIT[13]	Acute MI (6-40 days), LVEF ≤35%, HR ≥80 bpm, or SDNN average ≤70 ms	All-cause mortality	ICD vs. no ICD	In progress

Table 2 (continued)

Trial	Inclusion criteria	Primary end point	Study design	Primary results
IRIS[14]	Acute MI, NSVT>150 bpm, or HR >100 bpm at admission with LVEF <40%	All-cause mortality	ICD vs. no ICD	In progress
COMPAN-ION[15]	NYHA III or IV, at least 1 hospitaliza-tion, outpatient inotropes, ER visit in previ-ous 12 mo, QRS ≥120 ms and PR >150 ms, LVEF ≤35%, LVEDD ≥60 mm	All-cause mortality plus all-cause hos-pitalization	ICD with BiV, BiV vs. medical therapy	ICD w/BiV & BiV with lower all-cause mor-tality plus hospitalization compared with medical therapy

BiV, biventricular; bpm, beats/min; CABG, coronary artery bypass graft; CAD, coronary artery disease; CHF, congestive heart failure; CI, confidence interval; CMP, cardiomy-opathy; ER, emergency room; HR, heart rate; LVEDD, left ventricular end-diastolic dimension; LVEF, left ventricular ejection fraction; MI, myocardial infarction; NSVT, nonsustained ventricular tachycardia; NYHA, New York Heart Association; PVC, pre-mature ventricular complex; SAECG, signal-averaged electrocardiogram; SDNN, standard deviation of normal-to-normal heart beats; SDRR, standard deviation of RR interval; VF, ventricular fibrillation; VT, ventricular tachycardia.

*Results are preliminary. Data not published at time of manuscript preparation. Data from oral presentation by A. Kadish, American Heart Association Scientific Session, Orlando, Florida, November, 2003.

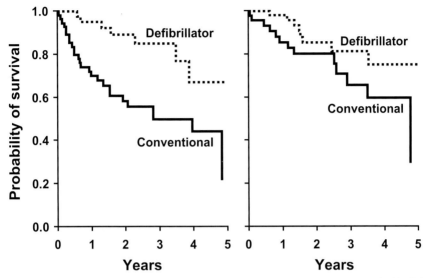

Figure 7. Survival curves from MADIT I post hoc analyses demonstrating survival by left ventricular ejection fraction. The subset of patients with the lowest left ventricular ejection fraction (<26%, left) had the greatest reduction in mortality. (From Moss AJ. Implantable cardioverter defibrillator therapy: the sickest patients benefit the most. Circulation 2000;101:1638-40. By permission of the American Heart Association.)

Similarly, in the MADIT II trial, patients in NYHA class I accounted for 35% of the ICD group and 39% of the conventional therapy group; those in class II, 35% and 34%; those in class III, 25% and 23%; and those in class IV, 5% and 4%, respectively, and 19% in the ICD group and 18% in the conventional therapy group had left bundle branch block. Of the 1,232 patients in MADIT II, 614 (50%) had a QRS duration of 0.12 second or greater. Although these primary prevention trials were invaluable in establishing the prophylactic role of ICD in patients with left ventricular dysfunction, the patients were not representative of those being considered for resynchronization therapy.

In MUSTT, patients with coronary artery disease, left ventricular ejection fraction of 40% or less, and asymptomatic ventricular tachycardia underwent electrophysiologic testing. Patients induced by programmed stimulation were randomly assigned to receive antiarrhythmic therapy, consisting of drugs and implantable defibrillators, guided by electrophysiologic testing, or no antiarrhythmic therapy. Patients whose treatment was guided by electrophysiologic testing had a lower incidence of cardiac arrest or arrhythmic death (25% vs. 32%). Patients receiving ICD therapy had the lowest incidence of cardiac arrest and arrhythmic death. The mortality at 5-year follow-up was 24% for patients who received the defibrillator compared with 55% for those who did not.

In MADIT II,[8] patients with coronary artery disease and a reduced ejection fraction (i.e., ≤30%) were randomly assigned to ICD or conventional therapy. Patients who had had a myocardial infarction within 1 month and coronary artery bypass graft surgery within 3 months were excluded. The mortality rate in the ICD arm was 14.2%, significantly lower than the 19.8% rate in the conventional therapy arm. The hazard ratio was 0.69 (95% confidence interval [CI], 0.51-0.93; P=0.016). There was a 31% reduction in the risk of death.

Ongoing studies, including the Sudden Cardiac Death–Heart Failure Trial (SCD-HeFT),[11] Defibrillators in Nonischemic Cardiomyopathy Treatment Evaluation (DEFINITE),[12] and Beta-Blocker Strategy Plus Implantable Cardioverter-Defibrillator (BEST-ICD), are examining the role of prophylactic ICD therapy in various patient populations and may be pivotal in establishing new indications for ICD therapy. The Comparison of Medical Therapy, Pacing, and Defibrillation in Chronic Heart Failure (COMPANION) trial is unique in that it involves combined ICD-resynchronization therapy and resynchronization therapy alone in a heart failure population (see below).

Clinical Trials of Combined ICD-Resynchronization Therapy

Many patients who are at risk for life-threatening arrhythmias may benefit from cardiac resynchronization (CRT)-ICD (CRT-D) therapy. Several clinical trials have examined CRT-D therapy,[19] including the CONTAK CD,[20,21] InSync ICD,[22] and COMPANION trials (Table 3). These trials have demonstrated the feasibility of combining the modalities of defibrillation and CRT. The COMPANION trial has most definitively demonstrated the importance of CRT-D therapy in a heart failure population.

The CONTAK CD trial[24] was conducted to examine the effectiveness of ICDs with resynchronization therapy. This multicenter trial was a randomized, parallel, double-blind trial that followed 581 patients with NYHA functional class II to IV (33% in class II, 58% in class III, 9% in class IV) heart failure, a QRS complex duration longer than 120 milliseconds, and an indication for ICD therapy. The mean follow-up time for the therapy phase of the study was 4.5 months and the mean duration of the implant was 13 months.

The CONTAK CD trial demonstrated that these more complex devices can be implanted at a high success rate. The success rate of the first attempt was 87%, with a perioperative mortality rate of 1.7%. In this study, CRT-D therapy was associated with a 23% decrease in mortality compared with that of a control group in which biventricular therapy was turned off. Also, hospitalizations for heart failure decreased 13%. The 21% decrease in progression of heart failure was not statistically significant.

Patients in the CONTAK CD trial demonstrated an increase in indices of cardiovascular function. Peak $\dot{V}O_2$ increased 0.9 mL/kg per minute compared with that of controls (P=0.003). Compared with controls, the 6-minute walk distance was 35 meters longer during CRT. The quality-of-life index increased by 16% for the CRT group compared with that of controls. For the subset of patients defined by NYHA class III and IV, left bundle branch block, and a QRS complex duration longer than 150 milliseconds, peak $\dot{V}O_2$ increased 1.9 mL/kg per minute compared with that of controls and the quality-of-life index increased 23%. Compared with controls, the 6-minute walk distance was 47 meters longer during CRT.

The InSync ICD trial[23] also examined a device that combined biventricular pacing with ICD capabilities. Patients were 18 years or older; had NYHA class II, III, or IV heart failure; a QRS complex duration of at least 130 milliseconds; left ventricular ejection fraction of no more than 35%; left ventricular end-diastolic dimension of at least 55 mm; heart failure that had been stable for at least 1 month;

Table 3. Cardiac Resynchronization ICD Trials

Trial	Inclusion criteria	Primary end point	Study design	Main findings
MIRACLE ICD[23]	NYHA II-IV, LVEF ≤35%, QRS ≥130 ms, LVEDD >55 mm, stable drug regimen ≥1 mo, ICD indication	NYHA class, QOL score, 6-min walk distance	CRT vs. no CRT	QOL score and NYHA class improved but no difference in 6-min walk distance; peak $\dot{V}O_2$ increased
CONTAK CD[21]	NYHA class II-IV, LVEF ≤35%, QRS ≥120 ms, ICD indication	Composite of all-cause mortality, heart failure hospitalization, and VT	CRT vs. no CRT	15% decrease in end point (P=0.35), peak $\dot{V}O_2$ increased, LV size decreased in CRT
BELIEVE	NYHA class II-IV, QRS >130 ms, LVEF ≤35%, LBBB, LVEDD ≥55 mm, ICD indications	LV-only pacing safe & effective, BiV ATP safe & effective	LV CRT + RV ATP vs. BiV CRT + BiV ATP	Enrollment completed

Table 3 (continued)

Trial	Inclusion criteria	Primary end point	Study design	Main findings
COMPANION[15]	NYHA class III or IV, at least 1 hospitalization, outpatient inotropes, ER visit in previous 1-12 mo, QRS >120 ms & PR >150 ms, LVEF ≤0.35%, LVEDD ≥60 mm	All-cause mortality plus all-cause hospitalization	OPT vs. CRT + OPT vs. CRT-D + OPT	CRT + OPT and CRT-D + OPT lower all-cause mortality plus hospitalization compared with medical therapy

ATP, antitachycardia pacing; BiV, biventricular pacing; CABG, coronary artery bypass graft; ER, emergency room; LBBB, left bundle branch block; LV, left ventricle; LVEDD, left ventricular end-diastolic dimension; LVEF, left ventricular ejection fraction; MI, myocardial infarction; NSVT, nonsustained ventricular tachycardia; NYHA, New York Heart Association; OPT, optimized pharmacologic therapy; QOL, quality of life; SAECG, signal-averaged electrocardiogram; VT, ventricular tachycardia.

angiotensin-converting enzyme (ACE) inhibitor or equivalent and β-blocker therapy for 3 months or more; and an indication for ICD. Patients were randomly assigned to biventricular pacing programmed "on" or "off" for 6 months. At 6 months, all patients had biventricular pacing programmed "on." The primary end points were quality of life (Minnesota Living With Heart Failure Questionnaire), NYHA class, and 6-minute walk. The primary end point was defined as being met if all three parameters achieved a significance at $P \leq 0.05$, if two parameters had $P \leq 0.025$, or if one parameter had a $P \leq 0.0167$.

A total of 639 patients underwent attempted implantation. Of these patients, 210 were in NYHA class II and 429 were class III/IV. Of the patients in NYHA class III/IV, 369 were randomized. The class III/IV patients were reported separately as planned before the start of the trial. Implantation of the resynchronization system was unsuccessful in 50 patients.

The InSync ICD trial was stopped when paired 6-month data became available for 112 patients in each group without crossovers or withdrawal. The study was closed for analysis on October 5, 2001. There were 182 patients in the control arm and 187 in the CRT arm. Fifteen deaths occurred in the control arm and 14 in the

CRT arm.   In this trial, therapy with biventricular pacing resulted in improved quality of life and NYHA classification.

Bradley et al.[25] have performed an extremely important meta-analysis of the CONTAK CD, InSync ICD, Multicenter InSync Randomized Clinical Evaluation (MIRACLE), and MUSTIC trials. These investigators found that resynchronization therapy was associated with a 51% decrease in mortality due to progressive heart failure compared with that of controls (Fig. 8). Resynchronization reduced hospitalization from heart failure by 29%, and there was a trend toward reduction of all-cause mortality. This analysis combined patients who received CRT-D therapy and those who received resynchronization therapy only.

COMPANION was the largest trial to examine the effect of biventricular therapy and CRT-D therapy on all-cause mortality and hospitalization. All patients had NYHA class III or IV heart failure; QRS duration of 120 milliseconds or longer; left ventricular ejection fraction of no more than 35%; left ventricular end-diastolic dimension of at least 65 mm; heart failure hospitalization for longer than 1 month but less than 12 months before enrollment; treatment of stable heart failure with diuretics, ACE inhibitor or equivalent, and spironolactone (1 month) with or without digoxin; and β-blocker therapy for at least 3 months. Patients were randomly assigned to optimal pharmacologic therapy; optimal pharmacologic therapy and biventricular pacing (CRT); optimal pharmacologic therapy, biventricular pacing, and ICD therapy (CRT-D). The primary end point was time to all-cause mortality or all-cause hospitalization. Secondary end points included all-cause mortality,

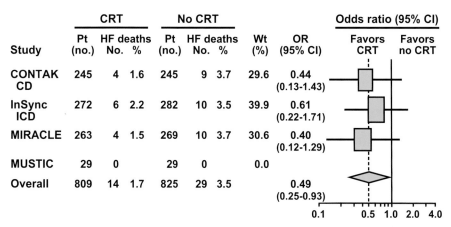

Figure 8. Odds ratio (OR) for CONTAK CD, InSync ICD, MIRACLE, MUSTIC, and the overall meta-analysis. Horizontal lines represent the 95% confidence interval (CI). CR, cardiac resynchronization; HF, heart failure; Pt, patients; Wt, weight given to each trial in statistical model. (From Bradley et al.[25] By permission of the American Medical Association.)

cardiac morbidity, maximal exercise (substudy), and others. Tertiary end points included submaximal exercise, quality of life, and others.

In the COMPANION trial, 1,520 patients in NYHA class III or IV were randomly assigned as follows: 308 to the optimal pharmacologic therapy arm, 617 to the optimal pharmacologic therapy and CRT arm, and 595 to the optimal pharmacologic therapy and CRT-D arm (Fig. 9). In each arm, 54% to 59% of the patients had ischemic cardiomyopathy.

The primary end point was reduced by 19% in both the CRT and CRT-D arms compared with the optimal pharmacologic therapy arm ($P<0.01$ and $P<0.02$, respectively). Similarly, all-cause mortality or hospitalization for heart failure was reduced by 36% and 40% in the CRT and CRT-D arms, respectively, compared with optimal pharmacologic therapy ($P<0.001$). All-cause mortality was reduced by 24% and 43% in the CRT and CRT-D arms, respectively, compared with the optimal pharmacologic therapy arm ($P=0.12$ and $P=0.002$) (Fig. 10).

This study highlights the benefit of biventricular pacing and biventricular pacing and defibrillation therapy in patients with heart failure of ischemic or nonischemic cause (Fig. 11).

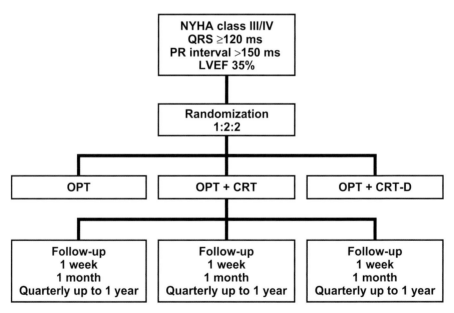

Figure 9. COMPANION design and randomization in the COMPANION trial. CRT, cardiac resynchronization therapy; CRT-D, cardiac resynchronization therapy plus ICD; LVEF, left ventricular ejection fraction; OPT, optimal pharmacologic therapy.[15]

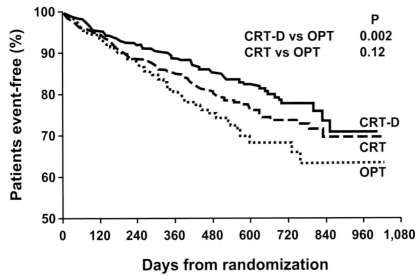

Figure 10. In the COMPANION trial, the secondary end point was all-cause mortality. In the OPT group, 12-month mortality was 19%. Mortality was decreased by 23.9% with CRT and by 43.4% with CRT-D. CRT, cardiac resynchronization therapy; CRT-D, cardiac resynchronization therapy plus ICD; OPT, optimal pharmacologic therapy. (From University of Colorado Cardiovascular Institute. COMPANION study late breaking trial slides. Available at: http://www.uchsc.edu/cvi. Accessed December 17, 2003. By permission.)

Selection of Most Appropriate Device Therapy for Heart Failure Patients: ICD vs. CRT vs. CRT-D

Does CRT Reduce Ventricular Arrhythmias and Obviate the Need for ICD?

Use of CRT has been shown to result in reverse remodeling of the left ventricle. In addition to its salutary effects on the neurohormonal system and ventricular hemodynamics, CRT has been hypothesized to reduce the incidence of ventricular arrhythmias. The important question extends beyond whether CRT reduces ventricular arrhythmias. The essential question is whether CRT reduces the risk of sudden cardiac death, obviating the need for ICD therapy. Garrigue et al.[26] considered, in a relatively early paper, the potential mechanisms by which CRT may reduce ventricular arrhythmias:

- CRT may alter the electrophysiologic substrate responsible for ventricular tachycardia in congestive heart failure—mechanism unknown

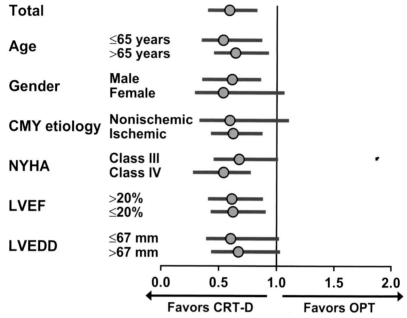

Figure 11. Subgroup hazard ratio from the COMPANION trial of CRT-D vs. OPT. CRT-D favored all subsets for all-cause mortality. CMY, cardiomyopathy; CRT-D, cardiac resynchronization therapy plus ICD; LVEDD, left ventricular diastolic dimension; LVEF, left ventricular ejection fraction; NYHA, New York Heart Association; OPT, optimal pharmacologic therapy. (Modified from University of Colorado Cardiovascular Institute. COMPANION study late breaking trial slides. Available at: http://www.uchsc.edu/cvi. Accessed December 17, 2003. By permission.)

- CRT may prevent reentry by reducing intraventricular conduction delay and dispersion of refractory periods to provide more homogeneous ventricular depolarization
- Inhibition of ventricular tachycardia may be enhanced by the proximity of the left ventricular lead to the reentrant site
- Improved hemodynamics may alter "stretch" that predisposes to reentry

Higgins et al.[27] observed that the incidence of ventricular arrhythmias recorded by ICDs decreased. Of 32 patients, 13 (41%) received appropriate therapy for ventricular tachycardia or fibrillation at least once in the 6-month period. Five patients (16%) had at least one tachyarrhythmic episode while programmed to biventricular pacing, 11 (34%) had at least one episode while programmed to "no pacing," 3 (9%) received therapy in both periods, and 2 received therapy with CRT only.

The authors summarized that although CRT may not obviate the need for ICD therapy, it appears to diminish significantly the number of appropriate ICD therapy episodes (antitachycardia pacing therapy and actual shocks).

Decreased ventricular ectopy has also been observed in comparing the absolute number after CRT with the absolute number before CRT.[28,29]

InSync (MIRACLE) provided a basis for comparing the incidence of ventricular tachycardia and fibrillation with and without CRT. Two patients in the "control" group had ventricular tachycardia or fibrillation that required treatment compared with six patients in the CRT group.

In InSync ICD, the absolute number of episodes of ventricular tachycardia or fibrillation was larger in the control group than in the CRT group (Fig. 12). However, the difference was not statistically significant, and the absolute number of episodes and the number of episodes per month were still substantial with CRT.

Selection of ICD Therapy for Patients With Heart Failure

For most patients with heart failure, the best approach is to determine whether the patient is a candidate for ICD and then assess whether the patient may benefit from resynchronization therapy (Fig. 13). As discussed above, the trials for primary and secondary prevention of ventricular arrhythmias included some patients with congestive heart failure, but this was not an entry criterion. Thus, most of these trials are not directly applicable to this patient population. However, because these trials have provided the best data available, we have only these data to rely on in determining the best treatment strategies.

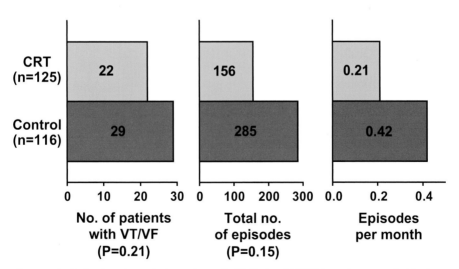

Figure 12. Episodes of ventricular tachycradia/fibrillation (VT/VF) in patients enrolled in the InSync ICD study—comparison of the control and active cardiac resynchronization therapy (CRT) arms.[23]

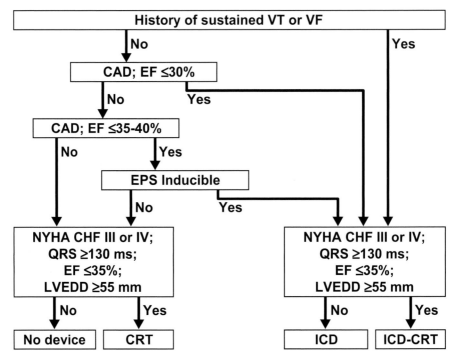

Figure 13. An algorithm to guide selection of ICD and/or CRT in patients with congestive heart failure. CAD, coronary artery disease; CHF, congestive heart failure; EF, ejection fraction; EPS, electrophysiologic study; LVEDD, left ventricular end-diastolic dimension; NYHA, New York Heart Association; VF, ventricular fibrillation; VT, ventricular tachycardia.

The COMPANION trial has provided some of the most relevant data about the use of ICDs and CRT-D in patients with heart failure. Unlike the primary and secondary prevention trials, patients were required to have been hospitalized for heart failure between 1 and 12 months before enrollment.

The indications for ICD implantation focus on two patient populations: 1) patients who have had a sustained ventricular arrhythmia or symptoms likely due to a ventricular arrhythmia and 2) patients at risk for ventricular arrhythmia. The American College of Cardiology, American Heart Association, and North American Society for Pacing and Electrophysiology guidelines classify the indications on the basis of the degree of agreement that the procedure is useful and the level of evidence (Tables 3 and 4). According to these guidelines, the approved indications for ICDs include the following (Table 5): cardiac arrest from ventricular tachycardia or fibrillation not due to a transient or reversible cause; spontaneous sustained ventricular tachycardia with structural heart disease or without structural heart disease not amenable to other treatments; syncope of undetermined origin with clinically

Table 4. Guidelines for Device Implantation

Class I: Conditions for which there is evidence and/or general agreement that a given procedure or treatment is beneficial, useful, and effective.

Class II: Conditions for which there is conflicting evidence and/or a divergence of opinion about the usefulness/efficacy of a procedure or treatment.

Class IIa: Weight of evidence/opinion is in favor of usefulness/efficacy.

Class IIb: Usefulness/efficacy is less well established by evidence/opinion.

Class III: Conditions for which there is evidence and/or general agreement that a procedure/treatment is not useful/effective and in some cases may be harmful.

Level of Evidence

Level A: Data are derived from multiple *randomized* clinical trials involving a large number of patients.

Level B: Data are derived from a limited number of trials involving a comparatively small number of patients or from well-designed data analysis of *nonrandomized* studies or *observational* data registries.

Level C: Consensus of expert opinion is the primary source of the recommendation.

For certain conditions for which no other therapies are available, the indications for device therapies are based on years of clinical experience as well as expert consensus and are thus well supported.

---

relevant, hemodynamically significant sustained ventricular tachycardia or fibrillation induced at electrophysiologic study when drug therapy is ineffective, not tolerated, or not preferred; coronary artery disease, previous myocardial infarction, left ventricular dysfunction (left ventricular ejection fraction ≤35%), nonsustained ventricular tachycardia, inducible ventricular tachycardia or fibrillation not suppressible with a class I antiarrhythmic drug; and coronary artery disease, at least 1 month after a previous myocardial infarction and 3 months after coronary artery revascularization surgery, left ventricular ejection fraction of no greater than 30% (based on MADIT II trial). These indications are described in greater detail in Tables 2 and 3.

For patients with heart failure, ICDs are particularly important because nearly half of the deaths of patients with heart failure are thought to be due to an arrhythmia, either tachyarrhythmia or bradyarrhythmia (Fig. 14).

The decision to implant an ICD in a patient with heart failure is based largely on risk stratification for sudden cardiac death. In addition, the patient's overall health and prognosis must be sufficiently good to warrant consideration of an ICD. Ultimately, the decision to implant an ICD is the result of weighing these considerations for the individual patient. For some patients with advanced heart failure

Table 5. 2002 ACC/AHA/NASPE Guideline Update for Implantation of Cardiac Pacemakers and Antiarrhythmia Devices: A Report of the American College of Cardiology/American Heart Association Task Force on Practice Guidelines (ACC/AHA/NASPE Committee on Pacemaker Implantation) ICD Indications

Class I
1. Cardiac arrest from VF or VT not due to a transient or reversible cause (*level of evidence: A*)
2. Spontaneous sustained VT in association with structural heart disease (*level of evidence: B*)
3. Syncope of undetermined origin with clinically relevant, hemodynamically significant sustained VT or VF induced at electrophysiologic study when drug therapy is ineffective, not tolerated, or not preferred (*level of evidence: B*)
4. Nonsustained VT with coronary disease, previous MI, LV dysfunction, and inducible VF or sustained VT at electrophysiologic study that is not suppressible by a class I antiarrhythmic drug (*level of evidence: A*)
5. Spontaneous sustained VT in patients without structural heart disease not amenable to other treatments (*level of evidence: C*)

Class IIA
   Patients with LV ejection fraction of less than or equal to 30% at least 1 month post myocardial infarction and 3 months post coronary artery revascularization surgery (*level of evidence: B*)

Class IIB
1. Cardiac arrest presumed to be due to VF when electrophysiologic testing is precluded by other medical conditions (*level of evidence: C*)
2. Severe symptoms (e.g., syncope) attributed to ventricular arrhythmias in patients awaiting cardiac transplantation (*level of evidence: C*)
3. Familial or inherited conditions with a high risk for life-threatening ventricular tachyarrhythmias such as long QT syndrome or hypertrophic cardiomyopathy (*level of evidence: B*)
4. Nonsustained VT with coronary artery disease, prior MI, and LV dysfunction and inducible sustained VT or VF at electrophysiologic study (*level of evidence: B*)
5. Recurrent syncope of undetermined origin in the presence of ventricular dysfunction and inducible ventricular arrhythmias at electrophysiologic study when other causes of syncope have been excluded (*level of evidence: C*)
6. Syncope of unexplained origin or family history of unexplained sudden cardiac death in association with typical or atypical right bundle branch block and ST-segment elevations (Brugada syndrome) (*level of evidence: C*)
7. Syncope in patients with advanced structural heart disease in whom thorough invasive and noninvasive investigations have failed to define a cause (*level of evidence: C*)

Table 5 (continued)

Class III
1. Syncope of undetermined cause in a patient without inducible ventricular tachyarrhythmias and without structural heart disease *(level of evidence: C)*
2. Incessant VT or VF *(level of evidence: C)*
3. VF or VT resulting from arrhythmias amenable to surgical or catheter ablation, for example, atrial arrhythmias associated with the Wolff-Parkinson-White syndrome, right ventricular outflow tract VT, idiopathic LV tachycardia, or fascicular VT *(level of evidence: C)*
4. Ventricular tachyarrhythmias due to a transient or reversible disorder (e.g., acute MI, electrolyte imbalance, drugs, or trauma) when correction of the disorder is considered feasible and likely to substantially reduce the risk of recurrent arrhythmia *(level of evidence: B)*
5. Significant psychiatric illnesses that may be aggravated by device implantation or may preclude systematic follow-up *(level of evidence: C)*
6. Terminal illnesses with projected life expectancy less than 6 months *(level of evidence: C)*
7. Patients with coronary artery disease with LV dysfunction and prolonged QRS duration in the absence of spontaneous or inducible sustained or nonsustained VT who are undergoing coronary artery bypass surgery *(level of evidence: B)*
8. NYHA class IV drug-refractory congestive heart failure in patients who are not candidates for cardiac transplantation *(level of evidence: C)*

LV, left ventricular; MI, myocardial infarction; NYHA, New York Heart Association; VF, ventricular fibrillation; VT, ventricular tachycardia.

and limited functional capacity, an ICD may not be appropriate because of limited overall life expectancy and quality of life.

Patients With Heart Failure and Reversible Causes of Ventricular Tachycardia

A reversible cause of a ventricular tachyarrhythmia decreases the risk of recurrence and is considered a class III indication for an ICD. For patients with heart failure and severe left ventricular dysfunction, the risk of recurrent ventricular arrhythmias is extremely high; therefore, most of these patients should receive an ICD. Because cardiac arrest alone may result in increased serum levels of creatine phosphokinase and troponin, patients who present with cardiac arrest and an increase in these cardiac markers are usually thought to be at continued risk for recurrent sustained ventricular arrhythmias. Therefore, these patients usually receive ICDs.

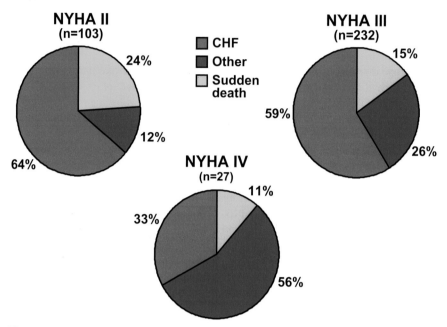

Figure 14. Modes of death by New York Heart Association (NYHA) functional class of patients enrolled in the MERIT-HF study. This study assessed the effect of metoprolol in congestive heart failure (CHF). (From MERIT-HF Study Group. Effect of metoprolol CR/XL in chronic heart failure: Metoprolol CR/XL Randomised Intervention Trial in Congestive Heart Failure [MERIT-HF]. Lancet 1999;353:2001-7. By permission of Elsevier.)

Syncope in Patients With Left Ventricular Dysfunction

Syncope in patients with left ventricular dysfunction and heart failure may be due to life-threatening ventricular arrhythmias and should be evaluated thoroughly. Both bradyarrhythmias and tachyarrhythmias may cause syncope. Other hemodynamic causes of syncope such as orthostatic hypotension due to excessive diuresis or low-output state should also be considered.

Clinical characteristics of the syncopal episode may help the physician assess the likelihood of a cardiovascular cause. For example, repeated presyncopal or syncopal episodes upon standing strongly suggest an orthostatic component rather than an arrhythmic cause. Syncope in a patient with left ventricular dysfunction, in the absence of strongly suggestive circumstances, should be considered potentially arrhythmic in nature. Because electrophysiologic studies have a relatively high sensitivity in the setting of coronary artery disease, many physicians use electrophysiologic testing to evaluate the potential risk of life-threatening ventricular arrhythmias. However, even in coronary artery disease, electrophysiologic testing does not have 100% sensitivity, and clinical judgment must be used to assess if an arrhythmic cause is likely. Because the sensitivity of electrophysiologic studies in patients with idiopathic dilated cardiomyopathy is even less than in patients with coronary artery disease, many physicians proceed to implantation of an ICD in patients with syncope and idiopathic dilated cardiomyopathy.[18] Many patients with left ventricular dysfunction and syncope meet the guidelines for ICD implantation on the basis of coronary artery disease and low ejection fraction alone (MADIT II criteria) or coronary artery disease, nonsustained ventricular tachycardia and inducible sustained ventricular arrhythmias (MADIT I criteria). These patients should receive an ICD on this basis in addition to their presentation with syncope.

Selection of Combined ICD-Resynchronization Therapy Device

Once the decision has been made to implant an ICD in a patient with heart failure, the indications for CRT should be reviewed. As stated elsewhere in this text, the current indications for CRT include class III or IV heart failure, widened QRS, and left ventricular enlargement and systolic dysfunction. Most patients who meet indications for both an ICD and resynchronization therapy should receive the CRT-D device.

Currently, the most difficult category is that of patients who meet the criteria for resynchronization but do not have a defined indication for ICD therapy. Patients with nonischemic cardiomyopathy are in this category. Currently, no randomized trials are specifically powered to examine this group of patients. The preliminary data from the COMPANION trial suggest that a mortality benefit was seen in patients with CRT-D compared with medical therapy alone but the upper limit confidence interval exceeded 1.0. Data from ongoing trials such as SCD-HeFT (Fig. 15) and DEFINITE (Table 2) may clarify the role of ICD therapy for patients with nonischemic cardiomyopathy, and the Defibrillation in Acute Myocardial Infarction Trial (DINAMIT) may clarify the role of this therapy for patients with acute myocardial infarction (Table 2). There may be an additional role for ICD and CRT-D as a bridge to heart transplantation, but the current guidelines do not include this indication.

Implantation of ICDs, CRT, and CRT-D Devices in Patients With CHF

Personnel and Experience

Personnel involved in implantation of ICDs and CRT-D in patients with severe heart failure and left ventricular dysfunction must have an extensive background in implanting devices in less severely ill patients. Criteria for training in implantation

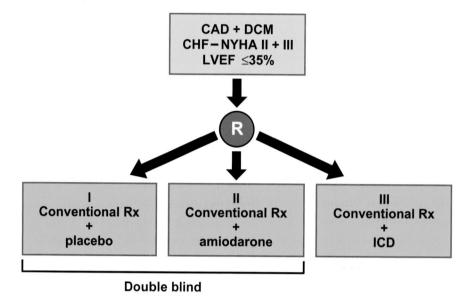

Double blind

Figure 15. Trial design for SCD-HeFT.[11] CAD, coronary artery disease; CHF, congestive heart failure; DCM, dilated cardiomyopathy; LVEF, left ventricular ejection fraction; NYHA, New York Heart Association; Rx, therapy.

of CRT and CRT-D devices have been published by the North American Society of Pacing and Electrophysiology.[30]

A patient with heart failure presents some of the greatest challenges at implantation because of the potential for severe hemodynamic instability and incessant ventricular arrhythmias as well as greater concern with renal function and implant-related use of contrast media.

Complications

Complications of ICD and CRT-D implantation in patients with severe heart failure may be more frequent when compared with recipients with less advanced heart failure. Potential complications that may occur during implantation are listed in Table 6. The risks of life-threatening complications may approach 1% to 2% in these patients, who may be particularly sensitive to sedation and not tolerate being supine without intubation. Also, worsening heart failure may develop during and after the implantation or the patient may have severe hypotension or cardiogenic shock. Implantation of a combined CRT-D device may increase the risk of renal dysfunction, potentially requiring dialysis, from the use of contrast agents for localizing the ostium of the coronary sinus and for coronary sinus venography.

Table 6. Possible ICD Implant-related Complications

Hemothorax
Pneumothorax
Damage to subclavian artery or vein, nerve plexus
Subclavian vein thrombosis
Superior vena cava syndrome
Cerebrovascular accident
Blood loss
Infection
Hematoma
Coronary sinus dissection
Lead dislodgment
Ventricular tachycardia or fibrillation
Atrial fibrillation
Atrioventricular block/transient bundle block
Need for electrical cardioversion
Burn to chest

Upgrade From a Preexisting Pacemaker

Many patients with heart failure may have a preexisting device. This subject merits discussion because the clinician may encounter patients with a preexisting pacemaker that warrants upgrade to an ICD/biventricular pacing device or a patient with an existing ICD that requires an upgrade to a biventricular pacing system. Such an upgrade will be affected by several considerations. One of the first considerations is the location of the pacemaker and the patency of the vein on that side. For a left-sided pacemaker with patency of the left subclavian vein, an upgrade on the same side may be quite straightforward. For a right-sided pacemaker, one must consider whether the pacemaker will be explanted and a new ICD will be placed on the left side. The advantage of using the left side is the potential for lower energy levels needed for defibrillation (defibrillation threshold). Alternatively, if the right subclavian vein is patent, the ICD may be upgraded on the right side. If the vein with the chronic pacing lead is occluded, the new device would most likely be placed on the contralateral side. (An alternative would be to extract the chronic pacing lead and reinsert new leads via the tract of the explanted lead. Technically, this is more difficult and would further prolong the procedure.)

The functionality and integrity of the pacemaker leads will determine whether they may be used in the new ICD to be implanted. The atrial lead may be used with the dual-chamber ICD system as long as the lead has the bipolar configuration. A bipolar ventricular lead could be used as the ventricular rate-sensing lead in the

ICD, but more commonly the lead would be capped and abandoned and a new lead placed for defibrillation.

An important concern in upgrading a pacemaker to an ICD is the potential for mechanical interaction, or "chatter," between the pacemaker and ICD leads, leading to oversensing. Positioning the ICD leads, often with active fixation, away from the preexisting pacemaker leads may prevent these problems.

The upgrade is potentially more challenging if upgrading to a CRT-D system. In addition to placing a new ventricular lead and positioning that lead in such a way to avoid interaction with the abandoned ventricular lead, the coronary sinus lead must also be placed. This requires that the vein being used can accommodate yet another lead. If the patient has a preexisting dual-chamber pacemaker, upgrading to a CRT-D system would mean a total of four leads in a vein unless the original ventricular pacing lead was extracted. At times, this can be accomplished and at other times, it cannot. In that circumstance, alternatives are limited. One option would be to place the new leads on the contralateral side of the chest and tunnel the newly implanted leads to the side of the chronic "pocket." The opposite could be done, and the chronic atrial lead that was to be in continued use tunnelled to the contralateral side and the device placed on the side of the new leads.

If the procedure is performed so that four leads are implanted via a single vein, there is concern about increasing the potential for symptomatic venous thrombosis. Although this usually can be managed with anticoagulation, the clinician and patient should be alert to this possible complication.

When a system is being upgraded, there is also potential for stenosis along the course of the chronically implanted lead, and this may impede the placement of the new lead or leads. An alternate venous approach may be required, for example, an epicardial approach or venoplasty.

Follow-up of Patients With Heart Failure Who Have ICDs and CRT-D

Coordinated Care

In the heart failure population with ICDs and CRT-D, it is critical that device follow-up be coordinated with follow-up for heart failure. It is essential that the personnel who perform these two forms of follow-up communicate about changes in the medical condition and new arrhythmia findings.

Recently, transtelephonic and wireless systems have been developed to aid in remote follow-up of patients with ICD and CRT-D. These advances will permit physicians to routinely obtain important data about episodes of arrhythmia and lead measurement, to evaluate ICD shocks, or to evaluate symptoms.

Evaluation of Heart Failure Parameters

ICDs and combination CRT-D have begun to provide information about the patient's activity and heart failure status. With an activity sensor, a plot can be made that illustrates the patient's physical activity and sensor activation. Incorporation of minute ventilation sensors may be particularly useful in following the patient's clinical status. Heart rate and heart rate variability may be of particular interest in tracking over time the patient's condition and autonomic state. Future devices will incorporate hemodynamic sensors that will enable caregivers to evaluate and adjust heart failure therapy (Fig. 16).

Future Directions

The previously described primary prevention trials such as MADIT I, MUSTT, and MADIT II have significantly increased the use of ICD therapy in patients with left ventricular dysfunction and coronary artery disease. Additional trials in progress, such as DEFINITE and SCD-HeFT, will further affect the use of ICD therapy. The

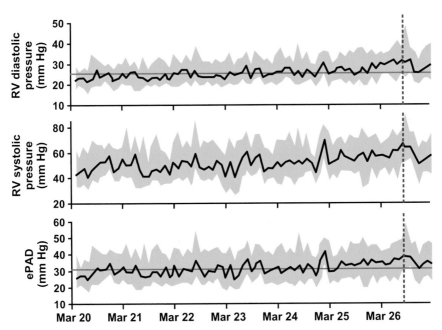

Figure 16. Hemodynamic trends of right ventricular (RV) diastolic pressure, RV systolic pressure, and estimated pulmonary artery diastolic pressure (ePAD) obtained from an implantable hemodynamic monitor. Although not yet incorporated in CRT-D, it is expected that subsequent generations of CRT and CRT-D will incorporate such features. (Courtesy of Medtronic.)

number of patients who are or potentially would be candidates for ICD therapy according to various clinical criteria and clinical trials are given in Table 7.

The COMPANION trial has demonstrated the importance of CRT and CRT-D therapy in decreasing mortality and hospitalization. The results of these resynchronization studies in combination with those of previous primary prevention ICD trials will lead to the widespread use of CRT-D devices in patients with heart failure. In the future, development of hemodynamic sensors will provide invaluable information for the follow-up of patients with heart failure. Incorporation of atrial therapies in ICD-resynchronization therapy may provide additional methods of treating atrial and ventricular arrhythmias in these patients.

A relevant and practical consideration for the future application of ICD and CRT-D therapy is cost. Cost and affordability will be important in the subsequent penetration of existing and future therapies.

The authors thank Dr. N. A. Mark Estes III for his review of the chapter and suggested changes.

Table 7. Projected Number of Patients Who Would Be Candidates for ICD Therapy Calculated by Various Study Criteria and by Country

Condition or study	Estimated no. of patients/ million	No. of patients			
		U.S.	Canada	Europe	Japan
VF/SCD	182	50,000	5,597	50,050	22,932
VT	727	200,000	22,355	199,925	91,602
MADIT/MUSTT	364	100,000	11,193	100,100	45,864
HCM + LQTS	220	60,500	6,765	60,500	27,720
MADIT II	2,455	675,000	75,491	675,125	309,330
SCD-HeFT	4,364	1,200,000	134,193	1,200,100	549,864

HCM, hypertrophic cardiomyopathy; LQTS, long QT syndrome; SCD, sudden cardiac death; VF, ventricular fibrillation; VT, ventricular tachycardia.

From Seidl K, Senges J. Worldwide utilization of implantable cardioverter/defibrillators now and in the future. Cardiac Electrophysiol Rev 2003;7:5-13. By permission of Kluwer Academic Publishers.

References

1. Swygman C, Wang PJ, Link MS, Homoud MK, Estes NA III. Advances in implantable cardioverter defibrillators. Curr Opin Cardiol 2002;17:24-8.

2. The Antiarrhythmics versus Implantable Defibrillators (AVID) Investigators. A comparison of antiarrhythmic-drug therapy with implantable defibrillators in patients resuscitated from near-fatal ventricular arrhythmias. N Engl J Med 1997;337:1576-83.

3. Kuck KH, Cappato R, Siebels J, Ruppel R. Randomized comparison of antiarrhythmic drug therapy with implantable defibrillators in patients resuscitated from cardiac arrest: the Cardiac Arrest Study Hamburg (CASH). Circulation 2000;102:748-54.

4. Connolly SJ, Gent M, Roberts RS, Dorian P, Roy D, Sheldon RS, et al., for the CIDS Investigators. Canadian Implantable Defibrillator Study (CIDS): a randomized trial of the implantable cardioverter defibrillator against amiodarone. Circulation 2000;101:1297-302.

5. Moss AJ, Hall WJ, Cannom DS, Daubert JP, Higgins SL, Klein H, for the Multicenter Automatic Defibrillator Implantation Trial Investigators. Improved survival with an implanted defibrillator in patients with coronary disease at high risk for ventricular arrhythmia. N Engl J Med 1996;335:1933-40.

6. Buxton AE, Lee KL, Fisher JD, Josephson ME, Prystowsky EN, Hafley G, for the Multicenter Unsustained Tachycardia Trial Investigators. A randomized study of the prevention of sudden death in patients with coronary artery disease [published erratum appears in N Engl J Med 2000;342:1300]. N Engl J Med 1999;341:1882-90.

7. Bigger JT Jr, for the Coronary Artery Bypass Graft (CABG) Patch Trial Investigators. Prophylactic use of implanted cardiac defibrillators in patients at high risk for ventricular arrhythmias after coronary-artery bypass graft surgery. N Engl J Med 1997;337:1569-75.

8. Moss AJ, Zareba W, Hall WJ, Klein H, Wilber DJ, Cannom DS, et al., for the Multicenter Automatic Defibrillator Implantation Trial II Investigators. Prophylactic implantation of a defibrillator in patients with myocardial infarction and reduced ejection fraction. N Engl J Med 2002;346:877-83.

9. Bansch D, Antz M, Boczor S, Volkmer M, Tebbenjohanns J, Seidl K, et al. Primary prevention of sudden cardiac death in idiopathic dilated cardiomyopathy: the Cardiomyopathy Trial (CAT). Circulation 2002;105:1453-8.

10. Strickberger SA, Hummel JD, Bartlett TG, Frumin HI, Schuger CD, Beau SL, et al., for the AMIOVIRT Investigators. Amiodarone versus implantable cardioverter-defibrillator: randomized trial in patients with nonischemic dilated cardiomyopathy and asymptomatic nonsustained ventricular tachycardia—AMIOVIRT. J Am Coll Cardiol 2003;41:1707-12.

11. Klein H, Auricchio A, Reek S, Geller C. New primary prevention trials of sudden cardiac death in patients with left ventricular dysfunction: SCD-HEFT and MADIT-II. Am J Cardiol 1999;83 (Suppl 5B):91D-7D.

12. Kadish A, Quigg R, Schaechter A, Anderson KP, Estes M, Levine J. Defibrillators in nonischemic cardiomyopathy treatment evaluation. Pacing Clin Electrophysiol 2000;23:338-43.

13. Hohnloser SH, Connolly SJ, Kuck KH, Dorian P, Fain E, Hampton JR, et al., for the DINAMIT Investigators. The Defibrillator in Acute Myocardial Infarction Trial (DINAMIT): study protocol. Am Heart J 2000;140:735-9.

14. Seidl K, Hoffmann E, Brüggemann T, Brachmann J, Andresen D. IRIS: Immediate Risk Stratification Improves Survival. Europace 2000;1:D293.

15. Bristow MR, Feldman AM, Saxon LA, for the COMPANION Steering Committee and COMPANION Clinical Investigators. Heart failure management using implantable devices for ventricular resynchronization: Comparison of Medical Therapy, Pacing, and Defibrillation in Chronic Heart Failure (COMPANION) trial. J Card Fail 2000;6:276-85.

16. Gregoratos G, Abrams J, Epstein AE, Freedman RA, Hayes DL, Hlatky MA, et al. ACC/AHA/NASPE 2002 guideline update for implantation of cardiac pacemakers and antiarrhythmia devices: summary article; a report of the American College of Cardiology/American Heart Association Task Force on Practice Guidelines (ACC/AHA/NASPE Committee to Update the 1998 Pacemaker Guidelines). J Am Coll Cardiol 2002;40:1703-19.

17. Winters SL, Packer DL, Marchlinski FE, Lazzara R, Cannom DS, Breithardt GE, et al. Consensus statement on indications, guidelines for use, and recommendations for follow-up of implantable cardioverter defibrillators. Pacing Clin Electrophysiol 2001;24:262-9.

18. Link MS, Costeas XF, Griffith JL, Colburn CD, Estes NA III, Wang PJ. High incidence of appropriate implantable cardioverter-defibrillator therapy in patients with syncope of unknown etiology and inducible ventricular arrhythmias. J Am Coll Cardiol 1997;29:370-5.

19. Cohen TJ, Klein J. Cardiac resynchronization therapy for treatment of chronic heart failure. J Invasive Cardiol 2002;14:48-53.

20. Bocchiardo M, Achtelik M, Gaita F, Trappe HJ, Lozano I, Higgins S, et al., for the VEN-TAK CHF/CONTAK CD Investigators. Efficacy of biventricular sensing and treatment of ventricular arrhythmias. Pacing Clin Electrophysiol 2000;23:1989-91.

21. Lozano I, Bocchiardo M, Achtelik M, Gaita F, Trappe HJ, Daoud E, et al., for the VEN-TAK CHF/CONTAK CD Investigators Study Group. Impact of biventricular pacing on mortality in a randomized crossover study of patients with heart failure and ventricular arrhythmias. Pacing Clin Electrophysiol 2000;23:1711-2.

22. Kühlkamp V, for the InSync 7272 ICD World Wide Investigators. Initial experience with an implantable cardioverter-defibrillator incorporating cardiac resynchronization therapy. J Am Coll Cardiol 2002;39:790-7.

23. Young JB, Abraham WT, Smith AL, Leon AR, Lieberman R, Wilkoff B, et al., for the Multicenter InSync ICD Randomized Clinical Evaluation (MIRACLE ICD) Trial Investigators. Combined cardiac resynchronization and implantable cardioversion defibrillation in advanced chronic heart failure: the MIRACLE ICD Trial. JAMA 2003;289:2685-94.

24. Barold HS. Preliminary clinical review of Guidant's Contak CD/Contak renewal heart failure devices and EasyTrak Lead System PMA. Available at: http://www.fda.gov/cdrh/panel/briefing/071001-tl-review.pdf. Accessed November 28, 2003.

25. Bradley DJ, Bradley EA, Baughman KL, Berger RD, Calkins H, Goodman SN, et al. Cardiac resynchronization and death from progressive heart failure: a meta-analysis of randomized controlled trials. JAMA 2003;289:730-40.

26. Garrigue S, Barold SS, Hocini M, Jais P, Haissaguerre M, Clementy J. Treatment of drug refractory ventricular tachycardia by biventricular pacing. Pacing Clin Electrophysiol 2000;23:1700-2.

27. Higgins SL, Yong P, Sheck D, McDaniel M, Bollinger F, Vadecha M, et al., for the Ventak CHF Investigators. Biventricular pacing diminishes the need for implantable cardioverter defibrillator therapy. J Am Coll Cardiol 2000;36:824-7.

28. Martinelli Filho M, Pedrosa A, Costa R, Nishioka S, Siqueira S, Crevleari E, et al. Biventricular pacing reduces frequency and complexity of ventricular arrhythmia in patients with congestive heart failure. Europace 2000:1 Suppl D:D227.

29. Walker S, Levy TM, Rex S, Paul VE. Biventricular pacing decreases ventricular arrhythmia [abstract]. Circulation 2000;102 Suppl 2:II-692-3.

30. Hayes DL, Naccarelli GV, Furman S, Parsonnet V, Reynolds D, Goldschlager N, et al. NASPE training requirements for cardiac implantable electronic devices: selection, implantation, and follow-up. Pacing Clin Electrophysiol 2003;26:1556-62.

CHAPTER 8

Future of Cardiac Resynchronization

David L. Hayes, MD
Paul J. Wang, MD
Jonathan Sackner-Bernstein, MD
Samuel J. Asirvatham, MD

The challenge in writing this text has been the incredibly rapid evolution of the field of cardiac resynchronization. This rapid evolution has been possible largely because of the ability to build upon the experience with other implantable cardiac devices.

As stated in the introduction and other places in the text, there are many unanswered questions, and despite the number of trials already completed, a number of investigations are still under way.

As we attempt to predict what the future may hold for cardiac resynchronization therapy (CRT), it seems reasonable also to consider "questions" that have not yet been answered satisfactorily. The questions that follow are ones we have asked or have been asked. Some of the answers are definitive and others are speculative. Some of the information that follows is covered in other portions of the text but represents issues of such clinical significance they bear repetition.

What Medical Therapies Hold Promise for the Near-term Future?

Several drug and biologic agents are in clinical development for the treatment of heart failure, both for the acutely decompensated state and for chronic disease. With the recent failures of anticytokine and antiendothelin agents, it is becoming increasingly clear that the ability to predict the success of drug therapies in development may not be much better than a coin flip. This is why all new therapies need to undergo rigorous testing and why we should not rely on smaller short-term mechanistic studies to shape practice patterns.

Should QRS Width Be Eliminated From CRT Implant Criteria?

As discussed in Chapter 2, important data have emerged that suggest ventricular dys-synchrony may exist in a patient with a narrow-surface QRS. We expect the surface QRS to be relied on less as a criterion. Instead, we will likely rely on an echocardiographic and Doppler-derived assessment of left ventricular dyssynchrony, as described in Chapter 6. However, studies will be needed to demonstrate improvement in quality-of-life indices, hospitalization for heart failure, and mortality.

Are There Better Methods to Select Patients for CRT and to Increase the Number of Patients Who Respond?

The use of techniques to assess the degree of interventricular and intraventricular dyssynchrony is likely to help select patients for CRT (see Chapter 6). However, it is still uncertain whether the response rate to CRT may be significantly increased using these techniques for patient selection and for optimization.

Should Patients With Right Bundle Branch Block Receive CRT?

Currently, data suggest that patients with right bundle branch block receive benefit from CRT if they meet the other criteria for CRT. The number of patients with right bundle branch block included in the randomized clinical trials is small. However, it appears that they received benefit equal to that of patients with left bundle branch block. As noted in other responses in this chapter, the degree of interventricular and intraventricular dyssynchrony as determined by echocardiographic Doppler techniques may be more important than QRS width or morphology.

If a Patient Is Hospitalized for CHF, and the Medical Regimen Is Optimized, Should CRT Be Considered Acutely?

Several databases establish that the first 3 to 6 months after discharge of a person hospitalized for heart failure is an extremely high-risk period.[1] If this is so and a device theoretically can reduce that risk, perhaps CRT should be considered during the initial hospitalization. This strategy may reduce the functional limitation of patients with heart failure. Obviously, the patient's condition must be stable enough to tolerate the procedure.

Will CRT Allow Tapering or Discontinuation of Medications?

The goal of CRT is to improve the quality of life after the medical regimen has been optimized. The goal of CRT is *not* to supplant or replace a medical regimen.

Medication dosage was assessed in an unpublished series of patients who had undergone CRT; diuretic therapy was subsequently reduced in a substantial percentage of these patients (Ritter P, personal communication, 2003). This observation is similar to that made in clinical practice when patients are "responders" to β-blocker or angiotensin-converting enzyme (ACE) inhibitor therapy. The mechanism is likely related to improved cardiovascular performance yielding better delivery of blood to the kidney, potentially reducing the requirement for diuretic therapy. In the Ritter experience, improved hemodynamics and pacing support allowed an increase in ACE inhibitor and β-blocker therapy.

Is There an Upper Age Limit for Considering CRT?

In the United States, when the fields of cardiac pacing and defibrillation and heart failure management are considered separately, therapeutic intervention (except for cardiac transplantation) is not usually decided on the basis of age. The decision whether to administer a particular therapy is usually decided on the basis of its potential benefit for the patient and the patient's functional and rehabilitative capacity. The same will likely be true for CRT.

Should CRT Be Considered in the Pediatric Population?

Clinical trials have been limited largely to adults. However, if a pediatric patient fulfills the accepted selection criteria, CRT should be considered. Permanent pacing and ICD systems are currently implanted in pediatric patients, with outcomes similar to those for adults. There are two other considerations in placing a CRT system in children. Because the long-term consequences of a coronary sinus lead are not completely understood, there is greater concern about placing this lead in a younger patient than in an adult. Also, a proportionally greater number of children who may meet the criteria for CRT likely have associated congenital heart disease. In many congenital anatomical disorders, variation in the coronary sinus and coronary venous system could make lead placement more difficult or impossible. For both these reasons, it may be more reasonable to accomplish cardiac resynchronization with left ventricular epicardial pacing.

Will We Ever Have Complete Resynchronization Therapy or Just Biventricular Pacing?

We typically use "resynchronization therapy" and "biventricular pacing" interchangeably, but they are not the same. Resynchronization of the ventricle is a noble goal, but we only get partway there with biventricular pacing. Synchrony is improved but generally not restored.

It appears that true resynchronization requires multiple leads placed across the left ventricle (and perhaps the right ventricle)—tasks difficult to achieve transvenously. The use of epicardial systems may be adequate to achieve resynchronization; however, because of the greater magnitude of such a procedure and the lack of ideal tools, it probably will be some time before we know whether epicardial systems will be more widely applicable for the purpose of achieving more "complete" ventricular resynchronization.

In addition to achieving less than complete ventricular resynchronization, "CRT" also may fail to achieve "cardiac" resynchronization in terms of ideal left atrial-to-left ventricular timing. It seems intuitive that atrioventricular timing may be better optimized by atrial septal or left atrial pacing (achieved either by coronary venous or epicardial access).

This experience will evolve from efforts to minimize episodes of paroxysmal atrial fibrillation by dual-site or alternate-site (septal) atrial pacing.

Is There a Role for CRT in Patients With Heart Failure Due to Diastolic Dysfunction?

This question probably should be qualified by whether the patient has systolic dysfunction as well. If the patient meets the current criteria for marked systolic dysfunction and also has diastolic dysfunction, CRT probably should be considered.

Because diastolic dysfunction is being identified as the cause of heart failure in a greater number of patients and therapeutic options remain somewhat limited, the potential role for CRT or left ventricular pacing in diastolic dysfunction has been questioned. Although early acute hemodynamic work by Kass et al.[2] in patients with left ventricular systolic function did not show a change in diastolic function with resynchronization therapy, the acute and chronic effects of resynchronization therapy in patients with isolated diastolic dysfunction have not been studied.

If CRT Is Beneficial for Patients in Class III or IV, Is It Reasonable to Hypothesize That CRT at a Less Severe Functional Stage (Class I or II) May Be Beneficial and Prevent Subsequent Development of More Severe Ventricular Dysfunction?

The ACC/American Heart Association classification of congestive heart failure describes disease progression from A to D, as shown in Figure 1. Currently, CRT is offered almost exclusively to patients with New York Heart Association (NYHA) class III or IV heart failure. These patients correspond to class C and D in Figure 1.

To date, CRT has consistently resulted in left ventricular reverse remodeling in randomized trials for patients in NYHA class III or IV. It is not unreasonable to assume that if CRT were applied earlier (i.e., asymptomatic or minimally symptomatic NYHA functional class I or II in the congestive heart failure classification), subsequent pathophysiologic sequelae would be minimized or avoided. This potential advantage is difficult to quantify relative to the small procedural risk.

Although previous trials included a small number of patients in NYHA class II, the data are limited. Ongoing trials are enrolling patients in NYHA class II, but it is not known whether a sufficient number will be included to determine how effectively disease progression will be limited.

There have been discussions about the application of CRT in patients in NYHA class I (class A in Figure 1). To our knowledge, no such trial has been initiated. Before advocating the use of biventricular pacing for healthier patients, the safety of device implantation, in addition to efficacy, needs to be evaluated in controlled trials.

Are Tools Available for Learning How to Cannulate the Coronary Sinus and to Place the Coronary Sinus Lead?

Models are available for manipulating a coronary sinus lead. They are of some value for becoming oriented to the anatomical location of the coronary sinus but are a poor substitute for the marked variations in the coronary sinus and coronary venous anatomy.

"Virtual" training models should be available in the near future. This type of model allows multiple variables to be programmed and the virtual coronary venous anatomy to be altered so lead placement may be made more or less difficult. This should be extraordinarily valuable for learning techniques for manipulating coronary sinus leads.

Physicians who are experienced in implantation but lack experience in the placement of coronary sinus leads should take advantage of the expertise of others. This expertise may come from electrophysiologists who routinely place leads in the coronary sinus and from coronary interventionalists. Coronary interventionalists may not cannulate the coronary sinus as often as electrophysiologists, but their experience in locating and cannulating the coronary arteries and established over-the-wire

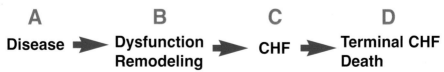

Figure 1. American College of Cardiology/American Heart Association classification (A-D) of congestive heart failure (CHF).

techniques can be valuable for others learning to locate, cannulate, manipulate, and respect the coronary sinus and coronary venous system.

Preoperative imaging techniques may aid in identifying the anatomy of the right atrium and the location of the ostium of the coronary sinus. Intracardiac transesophageal echocardiography, echocardiographic, and other real-time imaging methods may be used to help locate the coronary sinus.

Will the CRT Experience Lead to a Change in the "Usual" Pacemaker Implantation Technique for Patients Receiving Pacing Therapy for Standard Bradycardia Indications?

Experience with CRT has resulted in the development of coronary sinus leads that can achieve a stable position with reasonable chronic thresholds. If continued improvement of coronary sinus leads results in leads that can be positioned in the coronary sinus as easily and as safely as a lead can be placed in the right ventricle, a major shift in implantation technique is possible. Previous reports have assessed differences between right ventricular apical and septal or right ventricular outflow tract pacing.[3,4] Tse et al.[4] convincingly demonstrated a deleterious effect of right ventricular apical pacing. It is believed that they were able to demonstrate the difference between apical and outflow tract pacing because of a significantly longer follow-up period.

The Dual Chamber and VVI Implantable Defibrillator (DAVID)[5] trial and Mode Selection Trial (MOST)[6] both reported an increased risk of worsening heart failure associated with more frequent right ventricular pacing. On the basis of these data and the induction of left ventricular mechanical dyssynchrony caused by right ventricular pacing, it is not unreasonable to postulate that biventricular or left ventricular pacing could be advantageous. This needs to be tested in clinical trials.

Of course, there are no data about the long-term hemodynamic implications of left ventricular pacing in patients with normal left ventricular function. However, it seems reasonable to postulate that maintaining a more normal left ventricular activation pattern could negate the negative long-term consequences seen with the left bundle branch block activation pattern created by right ventricular apical pacing.

Who Should Perform Implantation of the CRT System? Is Specific Training Required?

Physicians who already have expertise in pacemaker and implantable cardioverter-defibrillator (ICD) implantation would be an obvious group to implant CRT systems. Despite experience with pacing or ICD implantation, the physician will still need to learn how to cannulate the coronary sinus and to place a left ventricular lead.

Guidelines for CRT implantation have been published recently.[7] Guidelines for training requirements to implant pacemakers, defibrillators, and cardiac resynchronization devices have been developed by the North American Society of Pacing and Electrophysiology (NASPE)-Heart Rhythm Society (HRS). The following levels of training have been defined: level 1, minimal exposure to implantable devices that can be achieved during most cardiovascular training fellowships; level 2, advanced training for a physician who desires expertise in device implantation without completing a full electrophysiology training program; and level 3, a fully trained electrophysiologist.

If cardiology training is intended to be inclusive of implantation of cardiac resynchronization devices, a physician with level 2 training would be required to participate as the primary operator in at least 15 CRT systems, including implantation of coronary sinus leads for left ventricular pacing. (This may include upgrades of existing pacemakers or ICD systems.) The trainee must have a thorough understanding of the principles of device management for congestive heart failure, including an understanding of coronary venous anatomy, electrocardiographic interpretation of left ventricular and biventricular pacing, the ability to interpret chest radiographs that include a coronary sinus lead, and an understanding of methods to optimize atrioventricular (AV) and ventricle-to-ventricle (VV) timing intervals following implantation of such a system.

If a physician expert in implantation of pacemakers and ICDs wishes to begin doing CRT implantations, he or she should also have a certain knowledge base and technical skills before beginning. No definite guidelines have been adopted by any professional society. However, it is likely that guidelines would include the following:

1) Observe a specific number of CRT cases in the institution of an experienced CRT implanter or implanting physician
2) Perform a defined number of CRT implants in the presence of an experienced proctor
3) Complete a didactic course in CRT with specified content which has been approved and endorsed by specific professional societies

These recommendations also apply to nonelectrophysiologists who are experienced and active in the practice of pacemaker and ICD implantation but who do not have experience in coronary sinus cannulation and coronary venous lead placement. If established standards (standards as defined by NASPE-HRS or the American College of Cardiology [ACC] or by the institution in which they work) require nonelectrophysiologists to have an electrophysiologist present or available to supervise defibrillation threshold testing, ICD programming, and follow-up during implantation of any device with ICD capability, these guidelines would also apply for implantation of a combined CRT-ICD device.

For any physician not actively engaged in implanting pacemakers or defibrillators (i.e., interventionalists, heart failure specialists, noncardiologists in an underserved area), the basic training guidelines in levels 1 and 2, namely, a training program, would have to be completed.

The safety and efficacy of epicardial leads for biventricular pacing have not been studied in large randomized trials. If transvenous coronary venous placement is unsuccessful, referral to a surgeon qualified to place an epicardial lead could be considered, but those training guidelines are not in the purview of NASPE. Training guidelines will need to be established for proposed methods designed for the nonsurgical placement of epicardial leads.

What Are the Long-Term Sequelae of Coronary Sinus Lead Placement?

The two issues that have been discussed most are late coronary venous thrombosis and concerns about coronary sinus lead extraction should the system become infected. To date, late coronary venous thrombosis has not been a concern; however, the total length of follow-up is relatively limited, so it may be too early to ignore this concern.

The extraction of leads from the right atrium and ventricle can be difficult, although newer extraction techniques with laser or electrodissection have markedly improved the success rate. Currently, the sheaths used for laser and electrodissection techniques are too large to be accommodated by the coronary sinus. Without a sheath of any kind that can enter the coronary sinus, extraction of the lead from where it enters the coronary sinus would be accomplished mainly by traction. Because of the relatively thin wall of coronary veins, there is concern that traction may cause the coronary vein to rupture or tear. Conversely, the design of current coronary sinus leads may make it easier to extract them (newer coronary sinus leads have a smaller French size and lack terminal fixation mechanisms such as "tines"). Still, the leads are designed so they are held against the wall of the vessel, and this point of contact would likely be a site of fibrosis.

Currently, our experience with extraction of coronary sinus leads is limited. A retrospective review from a center with a large experience with lead extraction reported on a total of 13 leads extracted from the coronary sinus. Four leads had been in place for less than 6 months and the other nine for more than 6 months. No serious complications occurred during the extraction procedure. One patient required autotransfusion during the extraction, and another subsequently was found to have thrombosis of the coronary sinus, which prevented reimplantation of the lead. The "usual" extraction tools were used, and the authors took great care as the dissecting sheaths got close to the ostium of the coronary sinus and they "limited" penetration of the sheath within the coronary sinus and kept the tip of the sheath away from the wall of the vessel. The authors hypothesized that the lack of serious complications might have been due partly to the angle at which the leads entered a peripheral coronary vein from the coronary sinus and also to the wall of the coronary sinus being tougher than the wall of the right atrium.[8]

With Newer Coronary Sinus Leads, What Is the Role of Epicardial Left Ventricular Stimulation?

Epicardial pacing should be considered in at least two situations. With current techniques for the placement of coronary sinus leads, there are some patients in whom a lead cannot be placed in a stable position. If the patient is thought to be an excellent candidate for CRT, epicardial pacing could be considered when placement of a coronary sinus lead fails. The patient should be assessed for surgical risk before undergoing epicardial lead placement. The right ventricular and atrial leads can still be placed transvenously either before or after the left ventricular epicardial lead has been placed. The surgeon can tunnel the epicardial lead to the prepectoral region where the CRT pulse generator is to be placed.

For patients with poor left ventricular function undergoing cardiac surgery (coronary revascularization or valve replacement), it may be reasonable to place a permanent left ventricular epicardial lead or leads at the time of the operation. If left ventricular function does not improve postoperatively, having the epicardial lead in place will simplify subsequent implementation of CRT.

Because of the beneficial acute hemodynamic effects of left ventricular and biventricular pacing,[9] if temporary epicardial pacing wires are to be used following a cardiac surgical procedure, it appears reasonable to place the temporary pacing wires on the lateral wall of the left ventricle instead of on the epicardium of the right ventricle. With this strategy, temporary pacing could become useful as a postoperative therapy for hemodynamic benefits, not merely for bradycardic complications.

Issues remain about the long-term function of epicardial leads. Historically, these leads have had a higher failure rate than transvenous pacing leads both in terms of fracture and higher thresholds. The development of platinized and steroid-eluting epicardial leads has resulted in markedly lower epicardial pacing thresholds. Still, epicardial leads are useful for CRT in some patients.

Is There a Role for Multifocal Right Ventricular Stimulation to Achieve Resynchronization?

There have been a number of investigations of bifocal or multifocal right ventricular stimulation for the purpose of cardiac resynchronization. However, to date, little material has been published. In the study of Pachon et al.,[10] leads were positioned in the right ventricular apex and right ventricular septum. Patients were then evaluated with septal versus right ventricular apical versus bifocal stimulation. Compared with conventional pacing, there was improvement in the ejection fraction, cardiac output, and peak filling rate; the QRS interval was shortened; and the left atrial size and mitral regurgitation area decreased, as did diastolic transmitral flow (E/A relation). Quality of life also improved significantly, with a score reduction of 50.4%. Bifocal stimulation demonstrated less significant improvement over septal stimulation only.

Additional data promote bifocal or multifocal right ventricular stimulation as a viable technique. The majority of these data have not been published and are not in the public domain. However, we believe that this is an idea that should not be abandoned. Depending on the tools that are developed and subsequent studies with this technique, it may be a viable approach.

Would There Be Incremental Clinical Benefit From a CRT Pulse Generator That Also Provided Hemodynamic Information Such as Pulmonary Pressure and Cardiac Output?

Information is available about chronically implanted systems for the purpose of monitoring pulmonary artery pressure. Measurement of cardiac output is also technologically possible. Several other intracardiac variables have also been measured as part of rate-adaptive pacing systems. These include peak endocardial acceleration, intracardiac impedance, preejection interval, dP/dt, and ventricular depolarization gradient.

Some of these variables may have added benefit in managing heart failure independently of how they could be used theoretically to autoregulate and hemodynamically optimize CRT. The added benefit in managing heart failure and autoregulating CRT would need to be weighed against the added cost to the device, the effect on device longevity, and the safety and reliability of another implanted sensor.

Are New Simplified Methods of Optimizing the Atrioventricular Interval and the Left Ventricular–Right Ventricular Offset Likely to be Developed?

Currently, several methods are available for optimizing the AV interval, including the use of echocardiographic formulas such as the Ritter formula, echocardiographic measurement of such variables as cardiac output, timing of pulmonary and aortic outflow, and hemodynamic monitoring techniques. Some clinicians have suggested using surface impedance methods to estimate cardiac output. Similar methods may be used to select the left ventricular–right ventricular offset.

Long term, it is likely that devices will be capable of auto-optimization of the AV and VV intervals. Data are emerging but are not yet available about the use of peak endocardial acceleration and other impedance sensors for antiregulation of the AV interval in CRT systems.

What Is the Longevity of a Biventricular Pacemaker?

A standard dual-chamber pacemaker generally lasts 5 to 8 years, depending on the percentage of time the patient is paced, lead impedance, and other factors. The current experience with chronically implanted biventricular pacemakers has not been long enough to know the actual longevity of the pulse generator. The manufacturers' estimates of longevity of current devices are shown in Table 1.

What Is the Current Reimbursement for CRT?

Under the inpatient prospective payment system (IPPS), Medicare sets the payment rate for a beneficiary's stay based on the Diagnosis-Related Group (DRG), which reflects the patient's diagnosis and the procedure performed.

The Centers for Medicare and Medicaid Services (CMS) has several established codes that apply to pacemakers and ICDs. CMS has created a new DRG for heart failure patients who require an ICD. CMS split DRG 514 (ICD implantation with coronary catheterization or electrophysiologic study) into two new DRGs so that patients with a diagnosis of acute myocardial infarction, heart failure, or shock receive higher payment because of the higher costs associated with these types of clinical problems. DRG 535 will be used for patients who qualify for an ICD, undergo cardiac catheterization or electrophysiologic study, and also suffer from heart failure, acute myocardial infarction, or shock. The new DRG provides higher reimbursement to hospitals for these patients than the DRG for non–heart failure patients who require an ICD, because of the increased resources needed to treat patients with heart failure. These payment changes help to support the added expenses related to CRT and combined CRT and ICD therapy.

CMS will now pay for CRT and ICD procedures coded with the combination of codes 37.95 (implantation of ICD leads only) or 37.97 (replacement of ICD leads only) and 00.54 (implantation or replacement of cardiac resynchronization defibrillator, pulse generator only) as total system implants under DRGs 535, 536, or 515 instead of DRG 115.

Table 2 summarizes the codes pertinent to CRT and combined CRT and ICD therapy.

Table 1. Projected Longevity of CRT Devices

Device	Volts	PW, ms	Other criteria	Ohms	Longevity, y
InSync 8040 (Medtronic)	2.5	0.5	DDR mode; 10% A pacing & 100% BiV pacing; 70 bpm	750 A 400 RV/LV	6.8
InSync III 8042 (Medtronic)	2.5 (A/RV) 5.0 (LV)	0.4	DDDR mode: 100% V pacing	600	6.9
InSync ICD 7572 (Medtronic)	4.0 LV & RV	0.4	Atrial tracking & 100% BiV pacing; 75 bpm	400	6.8
Marquis DR 7274	2.5	0.4	60 bpm, 50% pacing with biannual charges at 30 J	900	8.0
Marquis VR 7230	2.5	0.4	60 bpm, 50% pacing with biannual charges at 30 J	900	10.0
Renewal H 135 (Guidant)	3.5	0.5	DDD; 60 bpm; 15% A and 100% BiV pacing; quarterly shocks	700 RA/LV 900 RV	5.0
Renewal 3 H170 (Guidant)	3.0 RA 3.5 RV/LV	0.4 all leads	DDD; 60 bpm; 15% A and 100% BiV pacing; 6-14 shocks/ year at maximum of 31 J	700 RA/LV 900 RV	6.0
Renewal High Energy H177 (Guidant)	3.0 RA 3.5 RV/LV	0.4 all leads	DDD; 60 bpm; 15% A of 100% BiV pacing; 6-14 shocks/ year at maximum of 41 J	700 RA/LV 900 RV	5.0

A, atrial; BiV, biventricular; bpm, beats/min; LV, left ventricle; PW, pulse width; RA, right atrium; RV, right ventricle; V, ventricular.

Table 2. 2004 Hospital Inpatient Payment Rates for Selected DRGs That May Be Used With CRT or Combined CRT and ICD Implantation*

Procedure	DRG	Proposed 2004 average standardized reimbursement for large urban hospitals[†]
CRT-ICD system implant with EP or cath study	535[‡] = with AMI, HF, or shock	$39,265
	536[‡] = without AMI, HF, or shock	$30,186
ICD system implant without EP or cath study	515	$25,644
ICD lead or pulse generator implant or replacement	115	$16,986
Pacemaker or CRT implant	115 = with AMI, HF, or shock	$16,986
	116 = without AMI, HF, or shock	$11,299

AMI, acute myocardial infarction; cath, catheterization; CRT, cardiac resynchronization therapy; DRG, Diagnosis-Related Group; EP, electrophysiologic; HF, heart failure; ICD, implantable cardioverter-defibrillator.

*Applicable CPT codes include:

33208 = Insertion or replacement of permanent pacemaker with transvenous electrode(s), atrial and ventricular

33225 = Insertion of pacing electrode, cardiac venous system, for left ventricular pacing at time of insertion of pacing cardioverter-defibrillator or pacemaker pulse generator (including upgrade to dual-chamber system)

33249 = Insertion or repositioning of electrode lead(s) for single or dual-chamber pacing cardioverter-defibrillator and insertion of pulse generator.

71090 = Insertion of pacemaker, fluoroscopy and radiography, radiologic supervision and interpretation

[†]Payment rates are average standardized rates for large urban hospitals. Average payment rates for other hospitals will be slightly lower. Actual rates are often higher than average rates as the result of various add-on payments for individual hospitals.

[‡]In 2003, these services were under DRG 514.

References

1. Levy D, Kenchaiah S, Larson MG, Benjamin EJ, Kupka MJ, Ho KK, et al. Long-term trends in the incidence of and survival with heart failure. N Engl J Med 2002;347:1397-402.
2. Kass DA, Chen CH, Curry C, Talbot M, Berger R, Fetics B, et al. Improved left ventricular mechanics from acute VDD pacing in patients with dilated cardiomyopathy and ventricular conduction delay. Circulation 1999;99:1567-73.
3. Buckingham TA, Candinas R, Schlapfer J, Aebischer N, Jeanrenaud X, Landolt J, et al. Acute hemodynamic effects of atrioventricular pacing at differing sites in the right ventricle individually and simultaneously. Pacing Clin Electrophysiol 1997;24:909-15.
4. Tse HF, Yu C, Wong KK, Tsang V, Leung YL, Ho WY, et al. Functional abnormalities in patients with permanent right ventricular pacing: the effect of sites of electrical stimulation. J Am Coll Cardiol 2002;40:1451-8.
5. Wilkoff BL, Cook JR, Epstein AE, Greene HL, Hallstrom AP, Hsia H, et al., the Dual Chamber and VVI Implantable Defibrillator Trial Investigators. Dual-chamber pacing or ventricular backup pacing in patients with an implantable defibrillator: the Dual Chamber and VVI Implantable Defibrillator (DAVID) Trial. JAMA 2002;288:3115-23.
6. Sweeney MO, Hellkamp AS, Ellenbogen KA, Greenspan AJ, Freedman RA, Lee KL, et al., the MOde Selection Trial Investigators. Adverse effect of ventricular pacing on heart failure and atrial firillation among patients with normal baseline QRS duration in a clinical trial of pacemaker therapy for sinus node dysfunction. Circulation 2003;107:2932-7.
7. Hayes DL, Naccarelli GV, Furman S, Parsonnet V, Reynolds D, Goldschlager N, et al. NASPE training requirements for cardiac implantable electronic devices: selection, implantation, and follow-up. Pacing Clin Electrophysiol 2003;26:1556-62.
8. Tyers GF, Clark J, Wang Y, Mills P, Bashir J. Coronary sinus lead extraction. Pacing Clin Electrophysiol 2003;26:524-6.
9. Burkhoff D, Oikawa RY, Sagawa K. Influence of pacing site on canine left ventricular contraction. Am J Physiol 1986;251:H428-35.
10. Pachon JC, Pachon EI, Albornoz RN, Pachon JC, Kormann DS, Gimenes VM, et al. Ventricular endocardial right bifocal stimulation in the treatment of severe dilated cardiomyopathy heart failure with wide QRS. Pacing Clin Electrophysiol 2001;24:1369-76.

Index

Index note: italicized page references with an *f* or *t* indicate a figure or table on the designated page.